Unified Protocol
for Transdiagnostic Treatment
of Emotional Disorders
in Adolescents

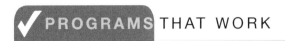

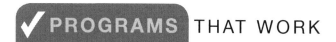

✓ PROGRAMS THAT WORK

TRANSDIAGNOSTIC PROGRAMS

Unified Protocol for Transdiagnostic Treatment of Emotional Disorders in Adolescents

WORKBOOK

JILL EHRENREICH-MAY

SARAH M. KENNEDY

JAMIE A. SHERMAN

SHANNON M. BENNETT

DAVID H. BARLOW

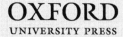

OXFORD
UNIVERSITY PRESS

OXFORD
UNIVERSITY PRESS

Oxford University Press is a department of the University of Oxford. It furthers the University's objective of excellence in research, scholarship, and education by publishing worldwide. Oxford is a registered trade mark of Oxford University Press in the UK and certain other countries.

Published in the United States of America by Oxford University Press
198 Madison Avenue, New York, NY 10016, United States of America.

ISBN 978–0–19–085553–6

9 8 7 6 5 4 3 2 1
Printed by WebCom, Inc., Canada

One of the most difficult problems confronting the parents of children with various disorders and diseases is finding the best help available. Everyone is aware of friends or family who have sought treatment from a seemingly reputable practitioner, only to find out later from another doctor that the original diagnosis was wrong or the treatments recommended were inappropriate or perhaps even harmful. Most parents or family members address this problem by reading everything they can about their children's symptoms, seeking out information on the Internet, or aggressively asking around to tap knowledge from friends and acquaintances. Governments and health care policymakers are also aware that people in need don't always get the best treatments—something they refer to as "variability in health care practices."

Now health care systems around the world are attempting to correct this variability by introducing "evidence-based practice." This simply means that it is in everyone's interest that patients of all ages get the most up-to-date and effective care for a particular problem. Health care policymakers have also recognized that it is very useful to give consumers of health care as much information as possible, so that they can make intelligent decisions in a collaborative effort to improve health and mental health. This series, Programs *ThatWork*™, is designed to accomplish just that for children suffering from behavioral health problems. Only the latest and most effective interventions for particular problems are described in user-friendly language. To be included in this series, each treatment program must pass the highest standards of evidence available, as determined by a scientific advisory board. Thus, when parents with children suffering from these problems or their family members seek out an expert clinician who is familiar with these interventions and decide that they are appropriate, they will have confidence that they are receiving the best care available. Of course, only your health care professional can decide on the right mix of treatments for your child.

This workbook is designed to help your adolescent learn to manage strong emotions more effectively and to overcome common life challenges. It outlines a program to better the lives of your adolescent and your family, and is most effective for teens around 13 years of age and above. This program was developed by some of the foremost experts on emotional disorders in young people, and has significant scientific support. The program is most effectively applied by working in collaboration with your teen's clinician.

Anne Marie Albano, Editor-in-Chief
David H. Barlow, Editor-in-Chief
Programs *ThatWork*

Accessing Programs *ThatWork* Forms and Worksheets Online

All forms and worksheets from books in the PTW series are made available digitally shortly following print publication. You may download, print, save, and digitally complete them as PDFs. To access the forms and worksheets, please visit http://www.oup.com/us/ttw.

Contents

Introduction to the *Unified Protocol for Transdiagnostic Treatment of Emotional Disorders in Adolescents: Workbook*

Welcome to Treatment!

Welcome to the *Unified Protocol for Transdiagnostic Treatment of Emotional Disorders in Adolescents: Workbook*! By starting this program, known as the UP-A for short, you have already taken a big step toward learning how to manage your emotions more effectively and how to overcome challenges in your life. This workbook will guide you through each week of the program with education, activities, and examples that will help you to better understand the role that emotions play in your actions every day. You will learn helpful strategies for dealing with uncomfortable emotions, and you will receive support in making choices that will move you closer to your long-term goals. We hope that you will learn a lot, challenge yourself, and maybe even have some fun! You may have questions about what the program is going to be like, what you will learn, and how you will feel. This introduction to the UP-A will hopefully answer many of your questions and will tell you more about what to expect from each part of the program.

A Note for Parents

This introduction may be helpful in answering your questions, too; however, the rest of this workbook is for your teen to use throughout the UP-A program. It will be up to your teen and his or her therapist to decide what will be shared with you from this workbook, but your participation is an important part of the program. Your teen's therapist will have separate handouts for you that are meant to accompany specific parts of this treatment.

We want you to learn the things your teen is learning so you can provide support and model effective strategies for handling emotions right along with your teen. The goal of this program is for everyone to become more comfortable tolerating and handling uncomfortable emotions. If your teen feels overwhelmed or tired in the beginning of this program, please talk with your teen's therapist about how everyone can work together to help your teen persevere. Over time, we expect your teen will be able to use more helpful strategies to manage emotions and decrease avoidance of appropriate and safe situations, places, people, and interactions that cause distress. Change doesn't happen overnight, and there are always good days and bad days, but making small, step-by-step changes each week will add up to positive, meaningful benefits by the end of this program.

Frequently Asked Questions

Who Is a Good Match for This Program?

Teens struggling with any difficult emotions (such as anxiety, sadness, irritability, anger, or fear) can benefit from this program. Here are some examples of young people who have participated in the program and some of the helpful changes they experienced.

> **Kate** is 16 years old and in the 11th grade. Before she started the UP-A, she put a lot of pressure on herself in school, drama, and choir, and always felt very anxious and upset if she messed up or made a mistake. She worried a lot about the future and what she was going to do after high school. Before starting the UP-A program, Kate was feeling down a lot and was arguing with others more easily, and her family said she didn't seem as happy as she used to be. She hadn't been enjoying doing things she used to really like, even during the summer when she was less stressed about school. Kate benefitted from something called emotion-focused behavioral experiments, where she added more enjoyable experiences into her day and followed through with doing these things even when she didn't feel like it. She also liked learning skills for challenging some of her unhelpful ways of thinking about her performance in school, drama, and choir.

> **Mike** is in the 10th grade and was on the swim team and basketball team. Before Mike started the UP-A, he worried a lot about his mother's well-being, and would become very anxious if he was away from her, especially if she didn't text him back right away. He would try to skip his away meets and games if his mom couldn't go, or he would call his mom repeatedly until she picked up. He would get very angry

at his mom, and would lose his cool with his friends more easily if he was worried or stressed out. This sometimes got him into trouble on the basketball court. Mike found it helpful to learn more about how his body felt when he was anxious or angry, and he was able to learn strategies for handling these sensations and emotions differently when he noticed they were building, without judging himself or getting mad at himself or others when something stressful was happening. He also challenged himself to go to all of his meets, games, and other school and social events, even if it meant he would be away from his mom, and he found this got easier over time.

Maria is 13 years old and in the 8th grade. She had obsessive-compulsive disorder (OCD), which means she had upsetting thoughts that repeated over and over in her head, and she spent a lot of time doing things to make herself feel better when she had these thoughts. Thinking these thoughts and doing these things were taking up a lot of time and getting in the way of having fun with her family and friends. Maria also sometimes pulled her hair out or picked at her pimples and had a hard time controlling these behaviors. Maria was a cheerleader and really liked math, and she sometimes felt like OCD was helpful because she believed that the behaviors of checking and rechecking her work or starting her cheer routines over again every time she made a little mistake prevented bad things from happening. At first, she was worried about changing these behaviors because she believed they helped her to perform better. However, Maria did a great job at becoming more aware of her thoughts, feelings, and urges in the present moment, and then she gradually stopped doing the behaviors and habits that were getting in the way of her life. She learned that she did not need to hang on to OCD to be great at the things that were important to her.

Kai is in the 9th grade and really struggled with making friends when he started high school. He was very anxious when meeting new kids and worried a lot about saying the right thing or embarrassing himself in front of others. He was teased and bullied in the locker room a lot and started trying to avoid going to school. He felt pretty depressed when he started the UP-A program and had missed several days of school. He found it helpful to learn a new strategy for solving problems more effectively. He learned to be more flexible in his thoughts about social situations and started worrying less about what other people thought, which helped him to be himself and make new friends.

These kids differed a lot from one another in what they liked to do, where they were from, and what was bothering them the most when they started the UP-A. However, they were alike in that they all struggled with managing their strong emotions and that their responses to their emotions were getting in the way of them being able to enjoy their lives. They all learned strategies for noticing, managing, and not avoiding difficult emotions, which allowed them to make more helpful choices.

What Can I Expect from This Program?

This program is a short-term one that is skills-based and requires practice. It may be different from therapies you have tried in the past. Your therapist will ask you to complete home learning assignments, which involve trying out new skills at home and reporting back during sessions. It is important for you to know that home learning assignments, as well as other worksheets and forms you will be using during sessions, appear at the very end of each chapter. The time spent on the skills in each section of this program is flexible and can be determined by you and your therapist together, depending on what is working best for you.

This program is broken down into eight chapters. Here is a brief overview of what to expect in each chapter. You can also check out Table I.1 for a quick idea of what is included in each part of the program.

Chapter 1: Building and Keeping Motivation

At the start of treatment, you will get to know your therapist and together you will identify what you hope to achieve by coming to treatment and participating in this program. Together with your parents and your therapist, you will decide on the top problems that you most want to change, and you will set realistic, achievable goals to work toward. You will also discuss what motivates you to keep participating in treatment, even when it feels really hard. These activities are typically accomplished in one or two sessions.

Chapter 2: Getting to Know Your Emotions and Behaviors

This chapter teaches you a lot of really important things about emotions. You may feel that you are already way too familiar with unpleasant emotions like fear, worry, sadness, or anger, but your therapist will try to help you think about emotions based on where they come from and what information they give you. You will come up with a way to label emotions, and identify the emotions that cause problems for you. You will also learn how to break emotions down into smaller parts as the first step for learning how you can use strategies to make your emotions feel more manageable. A really important thing you will learn about in this chapter is how strong emotions affect what you choose to do in certain situations. You will learn about what you do to try to AVOID feeling certain emotions, and how this may be causing problems for you. This information, and the worksheets that go along with it, will help introduce you to some of the most important terms and ideas in the entire treatment. Because of this, we typically spend two or three weeks making sure everyone understands and feels comfortable with the information, especially as it relates to you, your emotions, and your life.

Chapter 3: Introduction to Emotion-Focused Behavioral Experiments

In this chapter, you will learn about the connections between your emotions and behaviors (what you do), and practice some experiments to see if changing your behavior can affect the cycle of avoidance and your whole emotional experience. "Emotion-focused behavioral experiments" may sound a little weird before you really understand what they are. In these experiments you may be challenging yourself to do something even if you don't *feel* like doing it, which is a really important life skill as long as that thing is safe and helpful for you in the long run. Your therapist will first guide you through experiments involving the emotion of sadness, and will plan several activities with you that are associated with emotions like happiness, joy, and pride! You will likely spend one or two sessions on this chapter.

Chapter 4: Awareness of Physical Sensations

Chapter 4 focuses on learning more about what is happening in your body when you feel strong emotions, specifically the physical sensations (which we call body clues) associated with feelings like fear, anxiety, anger, or excitement. You will learn how to recognize clues from your body that provide information about emotions you are feeling and situations you are in. You will practice some exercises with your therapist that will bring up body clues safely, and your therapist will encourage you to respond to the body clues differently than you usually do. This chapter can take one or two sessions, or maybe more if this is something that is really important for you.

Chapter 5: Being Flexible in Your Thinking

In Chapter 5, you will focus on your thoughts and interpretations. You will learn how your brain allows you to do many things without thinking about them at all. Most of the time this is helpful, but sometimes your thoughts about situations are not accurate or helpful and can cause problems or make problems worse. In this chapter you will learn about the ways in which your emotions affect your thinking patterns, practice identifying your own unhelpful or unrealistic thinking patterns, and learn and practice strategies for coming up with different thoughts that are more helpful and/or realistic. You will also learn and practice strategies for solving some of the problems in your life more effectively. It takes practice to change unhelpful thinking patterns or problem-solving approaches into more helpful thoughts and problem-solving approaches, especially if you are used to thinking about things or responding to problems in a certain way. You will spend two or three sessions learning these skills but will continue practicing them throughout the rest of treatment and whenever you feel strong emotions!

Chapter 6: Awareness of Emotional Experiences

By Chapter 6, you will have learned a lot about emotions, and in this chapter you will really start to tune into your own emotions and experiences. You will learn how to become more aware of your emotions and the role your emotions play in your choices and what you do moment to moment. You will practice being more aware, less judgmental, and more accepting of your emotions and of yourself. You will likely spend one or two sessions on this chapter.

Chapter 7: Situational Emotion Exposures

Before really getting into Chapter 7, you will review everything you have learned in the previous chapters and will continue practicing the skills you have learned up to this point by planning and experiencing situations and things that bring up strong emotions. You will learn why it is important for you to gradually decrease your avoidance of uncomfortable emotions, whether this means facing your fears, fighting back against sad feelings, or handling your angry feelings in a more helpful way. You will make a plan with your therapist to gradually experience emotions you have been avoiding by changing your behavior step by step. You will practice these steps both in session and at home. Pushing yourself to respond to your emotions in a different way is hard work but also brings about lasting and rewarding changes. You may work out a plan with your therapist and your parents that includes getting rewards for your hard work, in addition to the very important rewards of solving problems and feeling good about yourself. This chapter is important and powerful for most people, so there is no limit to the number of sessions you might spend working on these goals. You will work this out with your therapist and parents.

Chapter 8: Keeping It Going—Maintaining Your Gains

By Chapter 8, you have worked hard and hopefully experienced the benefits of that hard work. You may have also had some fun or have positive feelings about what you have accomplished! It is time to celebrate your accomplishments and make a plan for the future. You and your therapist will review everything you have learned, and you will make a plan with your therapist for how to use your skills moving forward on your own.

You can also check out Table I.1 for a quick idea of what is included in each part of the program.

Table I.1. UP-A Program Summary

Chapter	Title	# of Sessions	What you will do and learn
1	Building and Keeping Motivation	1 or 2	▪ Get to know your therapist ▪ Share some things about yourself ▪ Discuss key problems and set goals ▪ Figure out what motivates you to change
2	Getting to Know Your Emotions and Behaviors	2 or 3	▪ Learn more about your different emotions ▪ Discuss why you have emotions ▪ Understand the three parts of an emotion ▪ Learn why you develop unhelpful actions
3	Introduction to Emotion-Focused Behavioral Experiments	1 or 2	▪ Learn about opposite action and emotion-focused behavioral experiments ▪ Track your mood and activity level ▪ Try making small behavioral changes and see what happens!

(continued)

Table I.1. Continued

Chapter	Title	# of Sessions	What you will do and learn
4	Awareness of Physical Sensations	1 or 2	▪ Learn about the connection between physical feelings and strong emotions ▪ Become more aware of your own physical feelings ▪ Start to do some exercises to bring up different physical feelings
5	Being Flexible in Your Thinking	2 or 3	▪ Learn and practice flexible thinking ▪ Learn common "thinking traps" ▪ Link thoughts to actions by using Detective Thinking and Problem Solving
6	Awareness of Emotional Experiences	1 or 2	▪ Learn and practice present-moment awareness ▪ Learn and practice nonjudgmental awareness ▪ Do a cool behavioral experiment using awareness strategies with emotional triggers
7	Situational Emotion Exposures	2+	▪ Do more behavioral experiments using exposure techniques ▪ Participate in exposures for situations that bring up the emotional behaviors that are a problem for you
8	Reviewing Accomplishments and Looking Ahead	1	▪ Review skills and progress toward goals ▪ Create a relapse-prevention plan
P	Parenting the Emotional Adolescent	1–3	▪ Build parents' awareness of responding to their teen's distress ▪ Introduce four common emotional parenting behaviors and their opposite actions (opposite parenting behaviors)

Why Do We Use This Approach?

As you can see in the examples we talked about earlier, there are differences in how strong emotions get in the way for each of us, but there is a common theme that makes many problems teens have with emotions and behaviors more similar than different. Many teens who participate in this program have trouble dealing or coping with strong or uncomfortable emotions, and their efforts to get rid of or control these emotions can make them act in ways that are not helpful to them in the long run.

This treatment can help you manage many types of tough emotions by providing a core set of skills that can be used to handle a variety of emotions and the unhelpful behaviors that have gotten in the way for you in the past and the present, and may continue to be problematic in the future.

This program is supported by research. That means that hundreds of other people, including many teenagers, have participated in this program before and have given a lot of information back to the authors about how well the program worked; what they liked about it; what they thought could work better; and what behaviors, emotions, or situations they were able to handle differently after completing the program. We followed many people for many months after they finished the treatment and discovered that most of them were still using the skills they had learned and were doing well!

When Should I Start, and When Can I Expect to See Changes That Will Be Helpful?

The sooner you begin working on how you handle your emotional experiences, the sooner things will start to get better. You will learn a lot about making choices when you feel strong emotions. While the choices you will learn to make may feel more challenging in the short term, they will make life much better in the long term. Many teens feel anxious or uncertain about starting this program, and they worry that it may take too much time away from other things. It's true that you may be giving up time after school in which you could be doing something else, but the time and energy you put into this program may end up allowing you to do even better in school and enjoy your other activities more as well. We think everyone should learn helpful strategies for managing difficult emotions as early in life as possible. Knowing how to deal with your emotions can even PREVENT problems from starting or from getting any bigger than they already are.

Practicing new ways to deal with strong emotions is hard work! At times during the UP-A program, you may notice that you feel worse before you feel better. This is understandable and normal. You may, for example, work on being okay while feeling anxious in order to learn how to cope with your anxiety, or you may work on letting yourself feel sad in order to learn how to cope with depression, and/or you may even practice experiencing your angry feelings and making good choices while in this state too. However, we do expect that if you complete this program and try to use the strategies discussed with your therapist, you should notice changes in the way you handle difficult situations and emotions by the end of the 12 to 18 sessions. Think about something that is four months from today. By committing fully to this treatment, you can expect that by that time, you will feel much better about your strong emotions and you will have learned new, more helpful ways to react to many of the challenges that brought you here.

This treatment will not always be easy. Your motivation for and commitment to treatment may go up and down at times, and that is normal and understandable. Change can be scary and hard, even if you know it is a good thing for you in the long run. While some teens do feel better each week, it is very common to feel better some weeks and worse during others. Ups and downs in your emotions and behaviors are a normal part of this treatment and, as long as you know to expect this, you will not feel too discouraged when you have a difficult week.

Where in My Life Will I Experience Helpful Changes?

Everywhere! Improving the way you notice, experience, and manage your emotions is related to positive changes in relationships with family and friends; your performance in school, work, or other activities; and how you feel about yourself. We are so glad you have taken this first step toward improving your life!

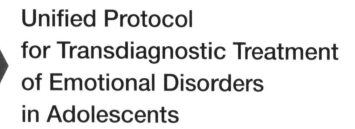

Unified Protocol
for Transdiagnostic Treatment
of Emotional Disorders
in Adolescents

GOALS

- To identify three top problems that you and your therapist will keep track of during treatment
- To identify three SMART goals based on your top problems
- To consider your motivation for coming to therapy and for working on emotions and behaviors that are not working well for you

Top Problems

This treatment is designed for teenagers who are experiencing feelings of sadness, anxiety, worry, anger, or other emotions that get in the way of their ability to enjoy their lives and feel successful. However, teens may differ a lot in the types of strong emotions that they are having and any problems these emotions seem to be causing them. For example, some teens with feelings of anxiety, anger, or sadness end up having problems like trouble making or keeping friends, conflicts with other kids at school, or trouble motivating themselves to go out and have fun with friends. Some teens may not have much trouble with friends but instead find that their emotions get in the way of their schoolwork. For example, their worry may cause them to procrastinate a lot, or they may struggle to participate in class. Strong emotions may also prevent some teens from joining clubs or activities, from going to parties, or even from leaving the house. Do any of these problems sound familiar, or are your top problems very different from these examples? Remember—this is *your* treatment, and you will get the most benefit from it by working on the problems that seem most important to you!

There are several reasons why we work with teens to create a list of three **top problems** at the beginning of treatment. First, identifying your top problems will help your therapist to make sure that he or she is creating in-session activities and home learning assignments that feel important to you. Second, identifying and rating how difficult your top problems are to manage will help remind you each week of goals that are important to you, and this may help you to stay motivated to work hard throughout treatment.

Additionally, in this treatment you may be asked to practice experiencing your strong emotions in a new way and may be encouraged to deal with situations in your life in a very different way than you are used to. *Talking about and experiencing your emotions may feel awkward or tough, especially at first.* When you understand how doing these things helps to solve your top problems, it will make them a little easier to do. Finally, you will be asked to rate each of your top problems every week on a 0-to-8 scale (from "not at all a problem" to a "huge problem"). When teens see that their ratings are starting to go down, and problems that used to feel huge seem much more manageable, it can be very exciting to know your hard work is paying off! Rating your top problems every week also helps you and your therapist know which problems to focus on and when to end treatment.

Your therapist will also be asking your parent about what he or she believes are your top three problems, and your parent will also be giving ratings for top problems every week. Sometimes, parents and teens agree about what the top problems are. However, sometimes they don't, and that is completely okay! Your top problems should be your own, even if your parent does not agree. Your therapist may also work with you and your parent to come up with a top problem list everyone feels comfortable rating together each week.

Sometimes, teens know exactly what their biggest problems are, but other times they don't. If you are struggling to come up with your three top problems, here are some questions you can ask yourself that might help:

- Is there anything I would like to see change in my life?
- What makes me think that I need to come to treatment?

- What does feeling fearful/worried/sad/angry stop me from doing or get in the way of?
- How would my life be different if I didn't feel so fearful/worried/sad/angry?
- How happy am I with my relationships with friends and family members?
- If someone offered to take one of my problems away, which one would I pick?
- What do my parents/friends/siblings/etc. think is my biggest problem? Do I agree?

Once you have identified your top problems, write them down on Worksheet 1.1: *Defining the Main Problems* (as a reminder, worksheets appear at the end of each chapter).

SMART Goals

Identifying the problem is just the first step. On Worksheet 1.1: *Defining the Main Problems*, you will also see that there is a space below each top problem to write a goal. If a *problem* is something that isn't going well in your life, then a *goal* is something that you work toward to help solve that problem. It is important to identify both problems and goals because goals help us to see ways of fixing or changing the problem and motivate us to take action!

Almost everyone understands the importance of setting goals, but not everyone knows that some goals help us to take action and to solve problems better than others. There are some common mistakes people make when setting goals, and it is important for you to know what those mistakes are so that you can avoid making them yourself. These mistakes include setting goals that are very vague or general, setting goals that make it hard to tell if you are making progress, setting goals that are very difficult or almost impossible to accomplish, setting goals that don't seem very important, and setting goals that take far too long to achieve or where the timeframe for achieving them is unclear. To help you avoid making these mistakes, think of the acronym **SMART goals** when you are setting each of your goals for treatment. A SMART goal is:

- **S**pecific: Specific goals are ones that are clear, concrete, and well defined. An example of a goal that is *not* specific is "doing better at school." A better, more specific goal is "raising my Algebra grade from a 'C' to a 'B'."

- ▤ **M**easurable: Measurable goals are goals that can be observed and tracked over time so that you can see how much progress you are making. An example of a goal that is *not* measurable is "making friends," because it is difficult to know whether you are making progress toward this goal. Have you achieved the goal if you made one new friend, or must you make more? A better, more measurable goal is "making three new friends."

- ▤ **A**ttainable: A goal that is attainable means a goal that you can achieve, or that is within your reach. Some goals are not attainable because they are very unlikely or because they are goals that a very, very small number of people could reach (for example, "become the Queen of England"). Other goals are not attainable because they would take a very long time to achieve, much longer than the amount of time you will be in treatment (for example, "get into a good college" if you are only 14). A better, more attainable goal is "raise my GPA from ___ last quarter to ___ this quarter."

- ▤ **R**elevant: A goal that is relevant is one that is meaningful to you and one that has something to do with the emotions that you will be focusing on in this treatment, such as fear, sadness, or anger. A goal that is not likely to be relevant to your treatment is "save enough babysitting money to buy a car." Although this may very well be a good goal, it does not have much to do with the emotions we will be focusing on in treatment. A better goal is "raise my hand once during every class, no matter how nervous I feel."

- ▤ **T**ime-bound goals are goals that are very specific about when and how often you would like something to occur. A goal that is not time-bound is "get out of bed in the morning." A better, more time-bound goal is "get out of bed when my alarm goes off each day for the next month."

Now that you know how to set SMART goals, identify one SMART goal for each of the top problems you identified previously. Write the SMART goals on Worksheet 1.1: *Defining the Main Problems.* You and your therapist can also think about what the first steps might look like in achieving your SMART goals, so you have a better sense of what kinds of changes to expect in this treatment.

After identifying their top problems and SMART goals, some teens may feel very motivated to begin making progress toward those goals by coming to treatment and completing in-session worksheets and home learning assignments. However, it is also very common for teens to feel unsure about whether they want to change things in their life right now. Even though you can identify ways your life might improve, you may feel overwhelmed about making changes and stepping outside of your comfort zone to do so. Some teens also have questions about whether this treatment will actually help them. It may be difficult at first to understand why discussing uncomfortable emotions and dealing with emotional situations differently will help you, especially if you have been struggling with strong emotions for a long time. After all, you might wonder why you would *choose* to put yourself in a situation that brings up feelings of fear, anxiety, sadness, or anger, when you could just avoid the situation and those emotions altogether. Some teens may also have doubts about treatment because they feel pressured to attend sessions by their parents or others, who they think may be overreacting or exaggerating problems. *You should know that all of these are completely normal reactions* to starting therapy, and it is okay to feel some or all of these things. And in the end, it is up to you to decide whether or not you want to make changes in your life.

Because it is so common for teens to feel uncertain or overwhelmed about making changes, it may be helpful to begin to think about the benefits and the costs of changing and not changing. In other words, when considering the benefits of no change, think about reasons why it may be good for things to stay the same. For example, maybe you won't have to deal with the possibility of rejection if you don't try to make new friends, or you will know that your mom is safe if you can call her all the time. Then, think about the costs of no change, or reasons why it's hard for things to stay the same. For example, maybe you'll continue to feel sad on the weekends if you don't make new friends to hang out with, or you'll keep feeling sick at basketball whenever mom is late. Next, think about the benefits of change, or reasons why it would be good for things to change. Maybe you'll enjoy school more if you have more friends to talk to throughout the day, or you will be able to do more with your friends if you're not calling your mom as much. Finally, think about the costs of change, or the reasons why it would be hard for things to change. Maybe starting conversations with kids at school you don't know will make you nervous, or you might worry more about mom at first if you don't know for sure that she is okay.

Use Worksheet 1.2: *Weighing My Options* to consider the benefits and costs of change versus no change. After you have completed the worksheet, look at what you've written down. Considering all the factors, does it seem worth it to make some changes? Are you willing to give it a try? We hope so! This workbook was designed for teens just like you to help them achieve their SMART goals and solve the top problems associated with strong emotions in their lives.

Worksheet 1.1: Defining the Main Problems

In this space, write down the main problems that are bringing you to treatment. Include things that bother you, as well as things that other people in your life think are a problem. These things could include feelings of intense sadness, anxiety, or anger. Problems could also include attitudes or behaviors that lead to getting in trouble, or things you do that might be harmful to you or others. *After identifying three "top problems," work with your therapist to identify a goal for treatment related to each problem or concern.*

1. _____

What is my goal? _____

2. _____

What is my goal? _____

3. _____

What is my goal? _____

Worksheet 1.2: Weighing My Options

When we think about making a change, it's sometimes hard to see all sides. We may ignore things we don't want to do or feel are too hard to do. Use the following worksheet to evaluate your choices and help you think through all the pros and cons of changing and not changing. Pick a behavior that you might consider changing and evaluate the costs and benefits of staying the same and the costs and benefits of changing. Use the example of Mike—who is weighing the pros and cons of changing how often he calls his mom to check on her safety—to help you fill out the form for yourself.

Benefits of NO change—Reasons it's good for things to stay the same:

Mike: I have a better chance of knowing my mom is safe if I call her all the time.

1. _____

2. _____

3. _____

4. _____

Costs of NO change—Reasons it's hard for things to stay the same:

Mike: I'll keep feeling sick at basketball whenever my mom is late.

1. _____

2. _____

3. _____

4. _____

Benefits of Change—Reasons it would be good for things to change:

Mike: I can do more with my friends and I won't bother my mom as much.

1. _____

2. _____

3. _____

4. _____

Costs of Change—Reasons it would be hard for things to change

Mike: At first I might worry more about my mom if I don't know for sure she is okay.

1. _____

2. _____

3. _____

4. _____

CHAPTER 2

Getting to Know Your Emotions and Behaviors

- To define common emotion words and identify which emotions you experience most often
- To learn about the purpose of emotions
- To learn about the three parts of an emotion
- To learn about the cycle of avoidance
- To practice breaking down your emotional experiences into their different parts

Identifying and Defining Your Emotions

There are many, many different words to describe emotions. You probably use or hear someone else use some of the most common ones—sad, happy, worried, angry—almost every day. Yet, how often do you stop to think about what exactly these emotion words mean? In order to know what we're feeling, and to describe what we're feeling to someone else, we must first understand the meaning of the words we use to talk about different emotions. Take a look at Worksheet 2.1: *Emotions I Have* (as a reminder, all forms will appear at the end of each chapter), which includes many of the most commonly used emotion words. See if you can define each emotion word listed. To help you with this task, here are some questions you may want to consider for each emotion word:

- What do you think it means to feel this emotion?
- When was the last time you felt this emotion?
- How did you know you were feeling this emotion?
- What were you thinking when you were having this emotion?
- Did you notice anything in your body when you were having this emotion?

As you move through the list of emotion words, also consider which emotions you experience most often and which you experience least often. Are there some emotions on this list that you experience many times every day? Are there any emotions you rarely experience at all?

The Purpose of Emotions

Think for a moment about what your life would be like if you never experienced emotions. What if you never felt happy, sad, angry, afraid, or worried? Would your life be easier? More difficult? What do you think would be different?

Most teens would probably agree that it would be nice to feel less angry, afraid, or worried. Since you are coming to treatment and working with your therapist to manage some of these feelings a little better, you probably feel this way too! However, even though these and other emotions often feel unpleasant, *emotions are normal, natural, and necessary for survival.* Emotions give us a signal that something is going on in our environment and we need to pay attention. The emotion does not want to be ignored because it is trying to tell us to do something important, like get away or get help. Many times, our emotions direct our behavior *automatically* so we don't have to spend time thinking about what to do. We call the thing the emotion is telling us to do the **emotional behavior**.

To illustrate emotions and emotional behaviors more clearly, imagine that you are walking to school and hear tires screeching. When you look up, you see that a car is speeding toward you and the sound is the driver slamming on the breaks in an attempt to stop the car. What emotion would you feel in this situation? What would your emotional behavior be? Many teens say that they would feel scared or afraid, and they would jump out of the way as quickly as possible. In this type of situation, your ability to feel fear is extremely important because it lets you know that something dangerous is happening, and it motivates you to figure out where the danger or the threat is coming from and try to avoid it. When there is something truly dangerous happening, fear is *normal, natural, and useful* in getting us to safety as quickly as possible.

Pleasant emotions, like excitement or happiness, also have a purpose. If emotions like fear or sadness are trying to make us *do* something to reduce the strength of the emotion, then emotions like happiness or excitement are trying to make us *do* something that will keep the pleasant emotion going. That might mean sharing our pleasant emotion with someone else, or continuing to engage in an activity that we really enjoy.

HOME LEARNING ASSIGNMENT

Using Worksheet 2.2: *Emotion Identification Practice*, choose two different emotions from Worksheet 2.1: *Emotions I Have* that you experience over the next week. Try to describe the purpose of each emotion, how you knew you were feeling the emotion, and the emotional behavior.

The Three Parts of an Emotion

When we talk about our emotions, it helps to think of them as having three parts:

1. **thoughts** (what we think);
2. **physical sensations** (what we feel in our bodies); and
3. **behaviors** (what we do).

You have already started to think about some of the behaviors associated with different emotions, and we will talk more about thoughts and physical sensations in just a minute. When you are having a strong emotion, however, you are probably not used to thinking about its three parts. For most people, strong emotions are often overwhelming and confusing. It can be helpful to think of strong emotions as "emotion twisters." Like twisters or tornados, strong emotions often form quickly, sometimes seeming to come out of nowhere. As you will notice if you turn to Figure 2.1: *Emotion Twister*, the thoughts, physical sensations, and behaviors whirl around quickly, blurring together. Sometimes when you are experiencing an emotion twister, you may not even be sure which emotion or emotions you are experiencing—you may know that you feel "bad," for example, but you may not be so sure about whether you are experiencing

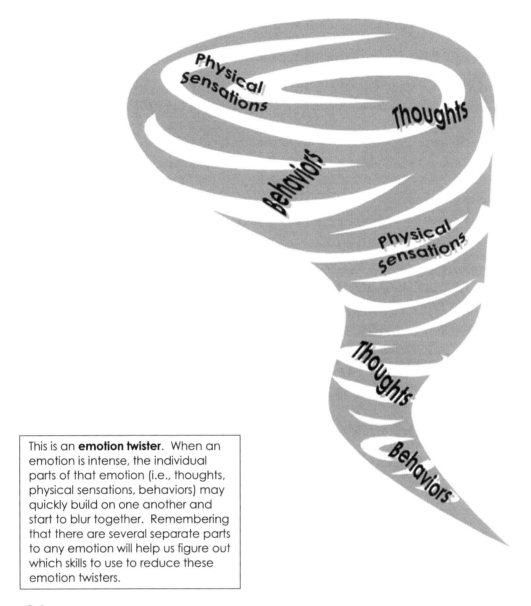

This is an **emotion twister**. When an emotion is intense, the individual parts of that emotion (i.e., thoughts, physical sensations, behaviors) may quickly build on one another and start to blur together. Remembering that there are several separate parts to any emotion will help us figure out which skills to use to reduce these emotion twisters.

Figure 2.1

Emotion Twister

anger, worry, sadness, or a combination of all three. Can you think of a time when you experienced an emotion twister like this?

Although you may sometimes feel like your emotions come out of nowhere, emotions always have a **trigger**. A trigger is something that causes the emotional experience. Sometimes triggers are easy to identify, such as performing poorly on a test or breaking up with a boyfriend or girlfriend. Other times a trigger may be a seemingly small event, such as hearing something on the news, seeing something, or hearing a comment from a friend or family member. A trigger might also be a physical sensation or a certain thought. To help you identify a trigger, it might be useful to use the phrase, "I feel sad/angry/worried because_____." Whatever comes after the "because" is usually the trigger. Can you think of any triggers that are tied to your emotional experiences?

Let's put it all together now. Once you experience a trigger, there are three parts to the emotional experience that follows (your thoughts, physical sensations, and behaviors). Each part of an emotional experience is connected to every other part, and the parts all interact and feed upon one another. To illustrate this, let's take an example. Pretend that it's Friday night, and you know you have to get your tooth pulled on Monday (**trigger**). You feel a bit worried and your anxiety begins to build. You start thinking about it even more over the weekend (**thoughts**), and the more you think about it, you start to feel nauseated (**physical feelings**). On your way to the dentist, you try to stall (**behavior**). This is a simple example of how the three parts of an emotional experience can impact one another.

This example describes a situation where your emotions build slowly over time. However, sometimes emotions can build up really fast. Imagine if you go to the dentist for a regular checkup and the dentist tells you, "I have to pull your tooth, and I can do it right now." You might feel afraid right away and think, "This is going to hurt; I don't want to do this" (thoughts). You might notice your hands getting sweaty or your stomach turning (physical feelings). You might look away or ask if there is really time to do the procedure that day (behaviors).

Whether the buildup is slow or quick, any of the three parts of the emotional experience can be involved. The more you focus on any one of these three parts, the more likely it will be to build upon and make the others stronger. As you saw in the *Emotion Twister*, when emotions are really strong, the individual parts might start to blur together. Remembering that they are separate parts and identifying those parts will help you figure out how to reduce your emotion twisters.

> **HOME LEARNING ASSIGNMENT**
>
> Turn to Worksheet 2.3: *Breaking Down My Emotions*, and try to think of one time during the past week when you experienced a strong emotion. Practice identifying the trigger and the three parts of the emotional experience.

Now that you have been thinking more about the different parts of your emotional experience—particularly your emotional behaviors—you may have noticed that you always choose to *do something* to manage your emotions. **Avoidance** is one strategy that may seem to work really well in the short term to temporarily get rid of the emotion, but that can actually make us feel worse in the long term. Can you think of a time you tried to avoid a trigger that was associated with a strong and uncomfortable emotion? Did that make you feel better? It might have. Often, when we avoid uncomfortable emotional experiences, we may feel better quickly. Because we learn that avoiding the uncomfortable situation makes us feel better, we may keep doing just that over and over again. The problem with avoidance is that we never learn that situations or emotions we feel are dangerous are not actually harmful, and they will pass on their own. We also never learn that we can experience strong emotions and tough situations but still get through them, without doing something to make them go away.

Let's take an example. Pretend that you are about to start a new project for school. The thought of beginning such a big task feels overwhelming, so you decide to put it off for a while. Putting it off might make you feel disappointed in yourself, but it helps you to avoid an even stronger feeling of being overwhelmed. The next day, when you have to go back to school, you remember the project and feel overwhelmed again. Your mind automatically thinks of just one way to feel better: doing the same thing that worked before, avoiding working on the project. While this may only make you feel better for a short time and may even mess things up in the long run, getting even a little relief from feeling overwhelmed may make you want to continue to avoid the project (in other words, may reinforce the avoidance).

Just knowing that avoidance does not help in the long run may be enough to help you stop avoiding what makes you feel uncomfortable. As well, you may be engaging in other behaviors you do not like (e.g., being mean or aggressive, going to sleep when you feel overwhelmed) that would also fit this same cycle or pattern that you will work with your therapist to identify as treatment continues. Overall, you will be learning other ways to respond to your emotions that will help you feel better both in the short term and in the long term during treatment.

We've now considered the role of triggers in your emotional experiences (the **before**). We've also explored the idea that your *responses* to those triggers (thoughts, physical sensations, and behaviors) interact to form your emotional experience (the **during**). Now, let's also think about the consequences of your choices (the **after**). We have just discussed the fact that when we choose to escape an emotional situation or avoid it altogether, we might immediately experience a feeling of relief in the *short term*. To go back to the dentist example, if you were to tell your dentist that you don't have time to have your tooth pulled today and will have to come back later, you would likely feel better right away. However, over the *longer term*, your tooth would still need to be pulled, and until the next appointment, you continue to feel anxious. The closer you get to the new appointment, the more you worry about how much it will hurt, and you begin to feel nauseated just thinking about your tooth. (You may also be feeling a lot of tooth pain by this time.) To go back to the **after**, even though you felt some immediate relief, you also experienced anxiety, worry, nausea, and tooth pain for many days until your next appointment.

As in this example, considering the before, during, and after of your emotional situations will help you begin to realize that while it may feel good to avoid emotional situations in the short term, avoidance usually has many unpleasant longer-term consequences. Understanding the before, during, and after of your emotions will help you change this cycle of avoidance and other emotional behaviors. Throughout this treatment, you will be tracking the before, during, and after of your own emotional experiences using Form 2.1: *Tracking the Before, During, and After* (at the end of this chapter).

HOME LEARNING ASSIGNMENT

Track the before, during, and after for at least one emotional experience over the next week, using Form 2.1: *Tracking the Before, During, and After.*

Worksheet 2.1: Emotions I Have

Below is a list of common emotion words. Some of these emotions may be very familiar while others are less familiar. While going through this list, think about which emotions you have experienced. How did you know that you were experiencing that emotion? What did you want to do when you were experiencing that emotion?

Anger	Fear	Pride
Happiness	Boredom	Shame
Anxiety	Embarrassment	Surprise
Sadness	Excitement	Jealousy
Joy	Hopelessness	Irritation

Worksheet 2.2: Emotion Identification Practice

Using Worksheet 2.1: *Emotions I Have,* choose two different emotions you experienced over the past week and use this sheet to describe them.

Emotion: _____

1. What do you think the purpose of_____is? Why do you think we have this emotion?

   _____

   _____

2. How did you know that you were feeling_____?

   _____

   _____

3. How did feeling_____make you act? In other words, did feeling

   _____make you do something that you might not have otherwise done?

   _____

   _____

   _____

   _____

Emotion:_____

1. What do you think the purpose of_____is? Why do you think we have this emotion?

   _____

   _____

   _____

2. How did you know that you were feeling_____?

   _____

   _____

   _____

3. How did feeling_____make you act? In other words, did feeling

   _____make you do something that you might not have otherwise done

   _____

   _____

Trigger:	**Emotions Experienced:**

Feelings in My Body

What I Do

What I Think

Form 2.1: Tracking the Before, During, and After

Each week, you will be asked to track the Before, During, and After of your emotional experiences. In order to change your emotional experiences, it is important that you understand the patterns that may occur (e.g., what triggers your emotional experiences, what happens as a result of your emotional experiences). This form will help you understand these patterns. By keeping this form and referring back to it later, you will start to see how changing one part of the pattern can change everything.

What happened Before? (What was the trigger?)	What happened During? (What was your emotional response to the trigger?)		What happened After? (What were the consequences of your emotional responses?)	
	Thoughts	Feelings	Behaviors	Short Term	Long Term

CHAPTER 3

Introduction to Emotion-Focused
Behavioral Experiments

GOALS

- To learn about the concepts of opposite action and emotion-focused behavioral experiments
- To learn about different types of activities and identify activities you enjoy
- To practice tracking emotion and activity levels and try a behavioral experiment for sadness
- To learn how to continue to do emotion-focused behavioral experiments

Acting Opposite: Introducing Opposite Action and Emotion-Focused Behavioral Experiments

In the next three chapters of this treatment, we will be focusing more closely on each of the three parts of an emotion, one at a time. In this chapter, we will concentrate on the behaviors part, or the thing that the emotion wants you to do. Look back at the *Tracking the Before, During, and After* form you have been completing for some of your emotional experiences so far. What behaviors did your emotions make you want to do, and what behaviors did you end up doing? Were what the emotion wanted to do and what you actually did the same, or were they different? If they were different, it's possible you may already be using one of the skills we will be discussing in this section: **opposite action**. Opposite action means noticing what the emotion wants you to do and acting in a different or opposite way.

Let's think about an example of an opposite action for sadness. Pretend you studied really hard for a test, and you ended up getting a grade that was much lower than you expected. Many teens in this situation would use words like "sad," "upset," "disappointed," or "down" to describe their emotions in response to this sort of trigger. If this happened to you and this was the way you were feeling, you might go home from school and spend the afternoon in your room, lying in bed and thinking about the test. You may not feel like talking to your friends or family. While it is completely normal to have these types of emotions in this situation, how do you think choosing to isolate yourself and continuing to focus on your grade would impact your emotions? Would it make you feel better? Probably not. In this situation, what do you think some opposite actions would be? Calling a friend, playing a game with your sibling, or even going for a walk are all examples of opposite actions in this situation.

In this chapter, you will be starting to practice using opposite action by doing what we call **emotion-focused behavioral experiments.** When scientists do experiments, usually they change one thing about a situation—while keeping everything else the same—and then look at the result. You will be applying this idea to an experiment with your emotions, which is why we call our experiments **emotion-focused**. We will be focusing on changing the emotional behavior or what you do in response to the emotion, which is why it is called a **behavioral experiment**. When we put that all together, we get **emotion-focused behavioral experiments**, which means changing our behavior and observing the impact on our emotions!

You will be working with your therapist in this chapter to do an emotion-focused behavioral experiment for the emotion "sadness" by acting opposite of what sadness wants you to do. We recognize that some teens may not struggle with strong feelings of sadness or depression, but if this sounds like you, we still think that the skills in this chapter could be helpful. Everyone has times in their lives when they experience strong feelings of sadness, and the skills in this chapter may be helpful during these times. Practicing an emotion-focused behavioral experiment for sadness will also help you to understand the concept of doing a behavioral experiment by acting opposite of what your emotion is telling you to do. Once you understand this concept, you can start applying it to other emotions as well. Talk to your therapist during this chapter about how to start using opposite action for other emotions.

Finding Activities You Enjoy

Many teens understand the connection between their emotions and activities, but when they are feeling depressed and down, it's hard for them to practice "acting opposite" by doing some activity. When nothing seems very much fun, it can be really difficult to think of an activity to do, and even more difficult to give your body enough energy to actually do it. This week, you will practice keeping track of your activities and trying, at least twice, to change your emotion by acting opposite of what your emotion wants you to do. If you have already created a list of activities you enjoy or that make you feel good, it is much easier to simply pick an activity from the list than it is to start figuring one out from scratch. Also, if you know that there are certain times when you are more likely to feel down or bored—maybe on Monday afternoons or on the weekends when you don't see your friends much, for example—you can make a plan to act opposite by choosing activities to do ahead of time.

When brainstorming activities to use as opposite actions when feeling bored or down, it can be helpful to think of examples of activities from five different categories:

- **Service activities** are activities that involve doing something that directly benefits or improves the lives of others, such as helping your sister with that project or volunteering at an animal shelter.
- **Fun activities** are activities that you enjoy and can do either on your own or with other people, such as painting or watching something funny.
- **Social activities** are activities you do with other people that are positive and fun, such as going out to see a movie with your friends or joining a club.
- **Mastery activities** involve learning a new skill or working toward becoming better at a skill, such as learning to bake or playing the piano.
- Finally, **physical activities** are activities where you get up and do something that involves moving your body, such as going for a walk or dancing around your room.

Think about the activities you do in a typical day and activities you do on the weekends. Are there things that you do because they make you feel relaxed, happy, excited, or energetic? Try to imagine that you have a day off from school with nothing scheduled. What would you do to have fun? What would make you feel like you accomplished something important to you? If you need help thinking of examples of activities you could do to improve the way you feel, take a look at Worksheet 3.1: *List of Commonly Enjoyed Activities* to come up with some ideas. Try to think of some activities from each of the five categories discussed above. You should also try to pick some activities that are very easy to do, that are cheap or free, and that you can do at home. Even just walking around your house or just outside of your house or apartment building can be a positive first step, if nothing comes to mind. Either way, try to write down at least a few activities on Worksheet 3.2: *My Enjoyable Activities List*. You can come back to this list from time to time as you think of new ideas for enjoyable, personally important, or valued activities.

Tracking Emotions and Activity During a Behavioral Experiment

Now that you have learned about the connection between emotions and activities and have started to identify activities you might enjoy, let's talk about how to use this information. Over the next week, you will be doing an emotion-focused behavioral experiment to see whether the number and type of activities you do on a daily basis have any effect on your emotions. You will be keeping a record for each day of your emotion level on a scale from 0 to 8 (the higher the number, the more relaxed, happy, excited, or energetic you feel), the number of activities you did, and which activities you did. Looking at these records at the end of the week will allow you to see the results of your experiment. You will be keeping your records in an emotion and activity diary much like Figure 3.1: *Kate's Emotion and Activity Diary*. What do you notice about the connection between Kate's emotional experiences and activities when you look at her diary?

Here is an example of an Emotion and Activity Diary that Kate has filled out for one week. The closer Kate's emotions are to an "8," the more relaxed, happy, energetic, or excited she is feeling. Use this example to help you fill out your own Emotion and Activity Diary on Worksheet 3.5.

Day of the Week	Emotion Level (0–8)	Number of Activities	Notes
Monday	4	5	Great day – tried out for a play at school and ate lunch with friends
Tuesday	2	3	Not as great – skipped choir to go home early after school
Wednesday	3	2	Boring day, not much to do, didn't hang out with friends
Thursday	2	1	Feeling really low, only got a small part in the school play
Friday	2	1	Just stayed home and watched TV
Saturday	2	1	More TV, really bored
Sunday	2	2	Mom made me go to mall with her, then went home and napped

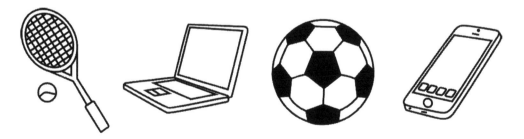

Figure 3.1

Kate's Emotion and Activity Diary

Many teens notice right away that Kate felt worse and rated her emotions lower on days when she did few activities, sat around and watched television, and did little socializing. Kate felt best and had the highest level of emotion on Monday, when she did the most activities, including spending time with friends and trying out for a play. Take a look at Figure 3.2: *Kate's Emotion and Activity Graph*, which clearly illustrates the connection between emotions and activity level. The dashed line is her daily emotion level rating, and the solid line is the daily total of quality, fun activities. As you can see, the lines tracking Kate's emotion level and activities tend to move up and down together. Kate's emotion level and the number of quality, fun activities are closely related. It's important to note here that the number of activities does not always need to be high for you (or Kate) to feel good. **Sometimes even one very exciting or enjoyable activity can decrease feelings of sadness and make you feel more relaxed, happier, or more energetic!**

The fact that Kate had a higher emotion level and felt particularly good on Monday probably means that she was excited about the possibility of

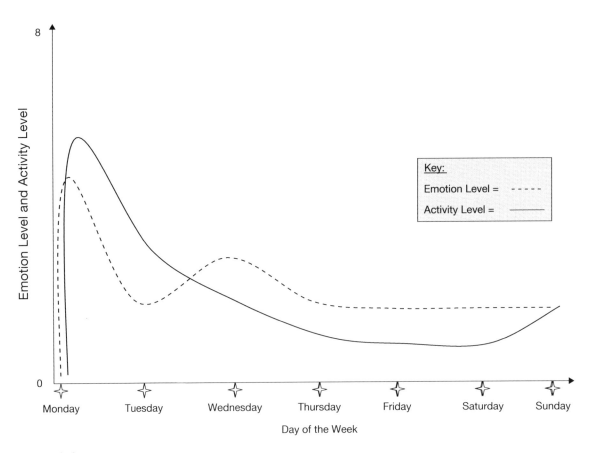

Figure 3.2

Kate's Emotion and Activity Graph

being chosen for the play and really wanted a part. What do you think Kate's emotions would have been like if she tried out for the play only because her friends were doing it and she really didn't enjoy acting? This likely would have resulted in Kate feeling worse and having a lower emotion rating on Monday. As noted, it is not just the number of activities we do that influences our emotions, but also the type of activities and whether they are enjoyable or important to us.

HOME LEARNING ASSIGNMENT

Over the next week, you will be completing your own emotion and activity diary and graph using Worksheet 3.3: *Emotion and Activity Diary* and Worksheet 3.4: *Emotion and Activity Graph*. Each day, look at the activities on Worksheet 3.2: *My Enjoyable Activities List*. Count up how many enjoyable activities you did that day, including activities on this list and any other activities you might have done. Write that total number in the box marked "Number of Activities" (on Worksheet 3.3: *Emotion and Activity Diary*) for that day. Please write down which activities you did in the "Notes" section. At the same time, you should also fill out your "Emotion Level" box on the worksheet, using the 0-to-8 scale provided. Remember that the higher your rating, the better you are feeling. If you notice any patterns or reasons for doing more or fewer activities, you can also write these in the "Notes" section. Remember—fewer activities may be just fine, as long as they are still improving how you feel. Use Worksheet 3.4: *Emotion and Activity Graph* to graph the lines for your emotion level and activities at the end of the week, just like Kate's.

Your second job this week is to pick two times to conduct an emotion-focused behavioral experiment by acting opposite of what your emotion is telling you to do. For example, if you notice yourself feeling sad or bored, pick an activity from Worksheet 3.2: *My Enjoyable Activities List* and try it out. Be sure to write down when you did your behavioral experiments by putting either a "Y" or "N" for each day in the column that asks, "Did I Try a Behavioral Experiment?" You may want to write about the experiment you did and how you felt afterward in the "Notes" section.

Emotion-Focused Behavioral Experiments: Keeping It Going

After recording your emotion level and activities for an entire week, now it is time to examine the results of your experiment. There are some common patterns that we often see when we look at emotion and activity diaries like the one you completed. Do any of these patterns apply to you?

High Emotion Level, High Activities

You did a lot of activities this week, and you felt consistently relaxed, happy, excited, and/or energetic. Great! One thing you may want to do is look at all the activities you did and consider how you were feeling during each of these activities. Did some activities improve how you felt more than others? Were your emotions different depending on whether you were doing mastery activities, fun activities, or social activities?

Low Emotion Level, Low Activities

You didn't do very many activities this week, and you had pretty low levels of happiness, excitement, energy, or relaxed feelings. If this pattern sounds like you, now is the time to think about acting opposite by introducing some new activities from Worksheet 3.2: *My Enjoyable Activities List*. If you didn't practice acting opposite last week, you may want to think about why. Did the activities seem too difficult or time-consuming, or require too much energy? If this is the case, you may want to pick short, small activities to start with. Think about taking some "baby steps" here before you work your way up to more intense or frequent activities. Sometimes changing activity levels can take a few weeks, and your therapist will be there to help guide you with this change.

Low Emotion Level, High Activities

You did a lot of activities this week, and your emotion level was consistently low. Let's think about why this might happen. Sometimes when we are trying to do too many activities in one day, we end up feeling overwhelmed, stressed, and anxious. Sometimes we may be doing a lot of activities but may not enjoy them because they don't feel meaningful, important, or enjoyable. Do either of these situations sound like yours? If so, you may want to think about either doing fewer activities or changing the types of activities you do to ones that feel more valued to you.

Some teens also find that an uncomfortable emotional experience or stressful event happened to them during the week, and as a result they felt worse and their activity level decreased a lot. If something like this happened to you, just noticing this pattern can help you to think about changing it in the future. Taking some time out for ourselves can be helpful when something stressful or emotional happens to us, but acting on this emotional behavior for too long can lead us to feel down or depressed.

HOME LEARNING ASSIGNMENT

If you tend to experience strong feelings of sadness or depression, or if you have found during your experiment that your activity levels are usually low, it may be helpful for you to schedule activities and track your emotion level on a more long-term basis. You can do this using Form 3.1: *Weekly Activity Planner*. At the beginning of each week, work with your therapist to plan and schedule some activities for each day. These activities can come from any of the five activity categories discussed in this chapter, or they could even be what are called **self-care activities**, like eating breakfast in the morning, doing your homework, or showering at night. At the end of each day, note which of the planned activities you actually did, the number of activities you did, and your emotion rating.

You and your therapist may also talk about how to act opposite for other emotions if you feel that you are not struggling with strong feelings of sadness or depression at this time. Your therapist can show you some materials from Chapter 7 to help support different types of opposite action.

As your therapist has discussed with you, each week you will be asked to track the Before, During, and After of your emotional experiences. In order to change your emotional experiences, it is important that you understand the patterns that may occur (e.g., what triggers your emotional experiences or what happens as a result of strong or intense emotions). Completing Form 3.2: *Tracking the Before, During, and After* this week can help you continue to learn about and understand these patterns. By keeping up with this form and referring back to it each week, you will begin to see how changing one part of the pattern can change everything. If doing both the Weekly Activity Planner and the Tracking the Before, During, and After forms feels like a lot more work than you can do in one week, please make sure to talk to your therapist about this so that he or she can tell you which form is more important for you to focus on right now.

Worksheet 3.1: List of Commonly Enjoyed Activities

Below is a list of activities (things to do, places to go, things to learn, etc.) you can try out to feel better by doing things you enjoy. Remember the five types of activities you learned about in session:

Service Activities – doing something directly for others or to improve the conditions of other people

Fun Activities – doing something that feels fun or exciting to you

Social Activities – doing something fun with others

Mastery Activities – doing something to learn a skill, working towards mastery

Physical Activities – getting up and doing some activity or playing a game

---

Try to choose activities from this list or come up with your own to see how your activity level affects your emotional experiences. Which of the categories above do these activities fall into?

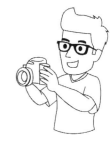

Visiting an aquarium
Going to an arcade
Art classes/projects
Babysitting
Playing Baseball
Shooting Hoops
Going to the Beach
Biking
Joining Book Clubs
Singing
Cooking
Doing Volunteer Work
Playing on the computer or tablet
Attending Concerts
Attending Church/Temple
Taking Dance Classes
Playing Field Hockey
Playing Football
Learning Foreign Languages
Grocery Shopping
Hiking/Taking a Walk
Meditating
Ice/Roller Skating
Playing Instrument
Knitting/Sewing
Playing Lacrosse
Playing Laser Tag

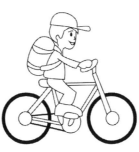

Doing Crafts
Watching Movies
Going to a Museum
Playing Paintball
Going to the Park
Taking Photos
Running
Drawing
Scrapbooking
Skateboarding Skiing/
Snowboarding
Learning Sign Language
Playing Soccer
Swimming
Playing Tennis
Writing
Yard Work
Doing Yoga
Going to the Zoo

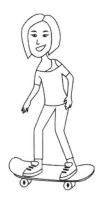

Think of your Own:

_____

_____

_____

_____

Worksheet 3.2: My Enjoyable Activities List

Use this chart to write a list of fun or pleasant activities. If you have trouble think-ing of fun activities, try imagining that you have a day off from school with nothing scheduled to do. What would you do to have fun, with no limits placed on you? Consider whether the things you think of are realistic, can occur regularly, and are positive choices, in order to help you generate your list of fun activities that you can track on your Emotion and Activity Diary.

	Name of Activity
1	
2	
3	
4	
5	
6	
7	
8	
9	
10	

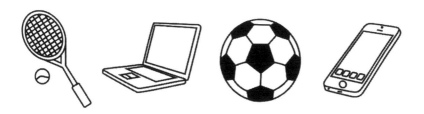

Worksheet 3.3: Emotion and Activity Diary

Here is an Emotion and Activity Diary for you to fill out. Use Kate's example if you need some help completing it. Remember that the closer your emotion level gets to an "8," the more relaxed, happy, energetic, or excited you are feeling. Try to record the number of activities you did each day, and use the "Notes" section to write down the types of activities you did. You should also note which days you tried a behavioral experiment this week. In the "Notes" section, you can also write down any changes you noticed in your emotional experience after doing the experiment.

Day of the Week	Emotion Level (0–8)	Number of Activities	Did I Try a Behavioral Experiment? (Y/N)	Notes

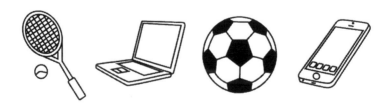

Worksheet 3.4: Emotion and Activity Graph

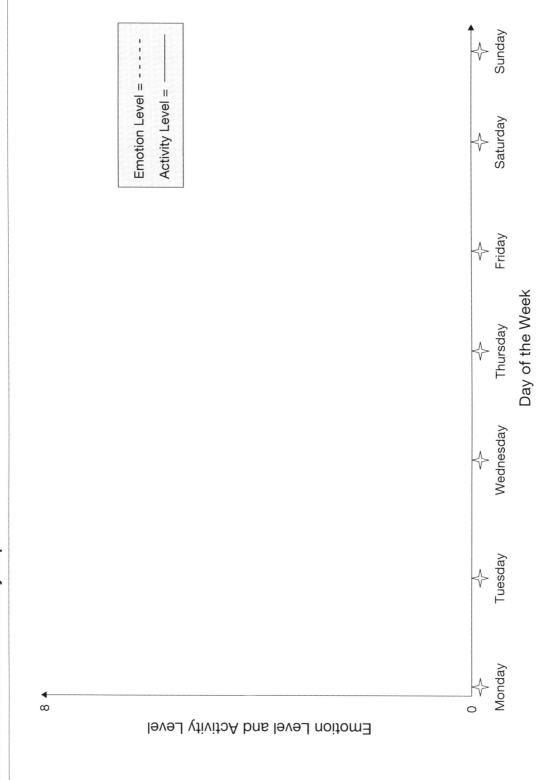

Emotion Level and Activity Level

8

0

Monday   Tuesday   Wednesday   Thursday   Friday   Saturday   Sunday

Day of the Week

Emotion Level = - - - - -

Activity Level = ——————

Form 3.1: Weekly Activity Planner

	MONDAY	TUESDAY	WEDNESDAY	THURSDAY	FRIDAY	SATURDAY	SUNDAY
Scheduled Activities							
Which ones I did							
Number of Activities							
Emotion Level							
Other Notes							

Form 3.2: Tracking the Before, During, and After

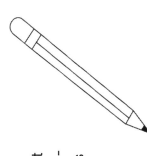

Each week, you will be asked to track the Before, During, and After of your emotional experiences. In order to change your emotional experiences, it is important that you understand the patterns that may occur (e.g., what triggers your emotional experiences or what happens as a result of your emotional experiences, etc.). This form will help you understand these patterns. By keeping these forms and referring back to them later, you can see how changing one part of the pattern can change everything.

What happened Before? (What was the trigger?)	What happened During? (What was your emotional response to the trigger?)		What happened After? (What were the consequences of your emotional responses?)	
	Thoughts	Feelings	Behaviors	Short Term	Long Term

CHAPTER 4

Awareness of Physical Sensations

- To learn about the connection between body sensations and strong emotions
- To use body scanning to become more aware of your body clues
- To practice experiencing your body clues without doing something to make them go away

Connecting Body Sensations and Intense Emotions

Think of a time when you felt a strong emotion. Maybe you were feeling anxious because you were about to give a presentation. Or maybe you were feeling angry because a friend said something mean to you or you got in an argument with your parents. Whatever your own experience with a strong emotion was, try to remember whether you felt any **physical sensations** in your body. This can be hard to do for many people, as we don't always pay attention to the feelings in our bodies unless they seem overwhelming (like when we are sick). But many teens would say that when they experience some of the emotions we have talked about in this treatment so far (e.g., happiness, sadness, anger, anxiety, fear), their body sometimes gives them a clue that tells them they are experiencing those emotions. So, let's call these **body clues.** For example, some teens report that their heart beats fast, or they feel sweaty and shaky when they are scared.

Interestingly, body clues may be part of something everyone's body does called **the fight-or-flight response**. This response sometimes happens at a time when something scary or sudden occurs, and our bodies respond in ways that allow us to fight off or flee the threat we perceive quickly. Some of the reactions our bodies have when we experience a fight-or-flight response include:

- Fast-beating heart
- Flushing or becoming pale
- A slowdown in digestion
- Tightening of muscles (caused by increased blood flow to those muscles)
- Shaking
- Sweating

The purpose of your body taking these quick actions is (1) to make sure enough blood gets to your muscles to take action if needed to protect yourself; (2) to supply your body with extra energy; and (3) to give you extra speed and strength—all to run away or fight off an attacker! The human body is pretty amazing in this way.

However, some teens feel these body clues even when their bodies aren't in danger and nothing is truly threatening. Part of our purpose in this chapter is to learn how your body reacts to such feelings of threat or concerns about harm and what to do if you notice these things at times when you are not truly in danger.

Sometimes the more strongly you feel body clues like these, the more you might think you are in danger (even if you are truly safe) and the more you might wish to get away from the situation you are in, contributing to that cycle of avoidance we talked about in previous chapters. At times, our body clues overwhelm us really quickly, and we may use an emotional behavior—like yelling or running away—to feel better as fast as possible, even though later that emotional behavior may not seem like best decision in the long term.

In the last chapter, we focused on changing one part of an emotional experience—our behaviors—in order to increase enjoyable activities in our lives and improve our mood. And, we also learned what an emotion-focused behavioral experiment was. In this chapter, we focus on increasing our awareness and ability to sit with another part of an emotional experience—our physical sensations—by conducting some different types of behavioral experiments. The purpose of these experiments is to help you to realize that, although body clues can be uncomfortable, they are not dangerous by themselves and will go away on their own. First, we will discuss the relationship between body clues and emotional experiences. Then, we will identify some body clues that you might have. Some people remember their body clues very clearly. For others, it is easiest to remember the body clues that they might have during emotional experiences if they conduct an experiment that makes them feel their body clues more clearly.

Using Body Scanning and a Body Drawing to Become More Aware of Your Body Clues

It can be fairly easy to identify your body clues in some situations. For example, when we go on a roller coaster, some of us feel emotions like excitement or fear, and experience body clues like a fast-beating heart, faster breathing, sweaty palms, or even nausea. During this chapter, you will be learning more about the body clues that you experience most often. However, it can be difficult to remember the body clues that you feel during more routine daily activities or even during experiences that bring up emotions such as happiness, anger, sadness, and anxiety.

Therefore, the first activity you will do in this chapter will help you to simply be more aware of the body clues you can sense during different types of emotional experiences or at other times when your body is feeling strong sensations. Your therapist will lead you through an activity called **body scanning**, which involves paying very close attention and purposely noticing any feelings you may have in your body. Your therapist will have you notice one part of your body at a time, starting with your head and slowly working your attention all the way down to your toes. The purpose of doing this is to increase your awareness of any body clues that you are experiencing currently, and also to help you remember body clues that you have felt recently during emotional experiences. Then, your therapist will ask you to try to write down or illustrate some of the body clues that you have noticed during emotional experiences using Worksheet 4.1: *Body Drawing*. Body clues tell us important information about emotions, but everyone experiences emotions and body clues differently! As you write down or illustrate your body clues, think about the emotions that you experience most often or most strongly, and try to think of at least a few body clues that accompany different emotional experiences.

For example, what you feel in your body may be different if you are sad versus angry or happy!

Think about the body clues that you wrote down or illustrated on your body drawing. Do these body clues feel good or do they make you feel uncomfortable? Can that change depending on where you are or what you are doing when you experience them? Do they make you want to do something, such as avoid the situation or trigger that is bringing on the body clues?

Experiencing Your Body Clues

The body clues you notice either during an emotional experience or during other activities, as long as you are in a safe situation, are normal, natural, and are not harmful—even if they DO feel intense or overwhelming at times. In order to demonstrate this, you and your therapist will conduct an experiment that is meant to make you feel physical sensations similar to those that you might feel when you are experiencing a strong emotion.

By conducting some experiments that make us feel the same sensations that we feel when we are experiencing strong emotions, we can teach ourselves that the body clues that we experience are normal and natural and cannot harm us. We call these experiments **sensational exposures**. Below is a list of possible sensational exposures that you and your therapist may try out together or that your therapist may assign for home learning:

- Shake your head side to side for 30 seconds.
- Run in place for 1 minute.
- Hold your breath for 30 seconds.
- Spin in a chair for 1 minute.
- Breath through a thin straw for 2 minutes while holding your nose closed.
- Hold a push-up position for as long as possible.

After you complete each sensational exposure, use the body scanning technique you have learned to pay attention to your body clues without trying to avoid or distract from them. How did it feel in your body and emotionally to complete this exercise? How did the sensations change over time? Use Worksheet 4.2: *Monitoring How My Body Feels* to track how you respond to each of these tasks.

Some teens will notice that the body clues they have when doing these experiments are uncomfortable at first and remind them of body clues that they have experienced during strong emotions such as anxiety, fear, anger, or sadness. These sensations should and will go away on their own, but it may take a bit of time. The more you practice these sensational exposures while noticing your body clues and reminding yourself that they're not dangerous, the less these physical sensations will bother you over time, and the less they will impact your emotions.

HOME LEARNING ASSIGNMENT

Over the next week, you will complete several more sensational exposures on your own at home. These sensational exposures might cause you to feel body clues that are similar to those you have during your emotional experiences. You may use either Form 4.1: *Tracking the Before, During, and After* or Worksheet 4.2: *Monitoring How My Body Feels* to track which sensational exposures you complete and anything you might notice about your thoughts, feelings, and behaviors while completing them. Remember, as you and your therapist might have discussed, it is important not to do anything to make these sensations go away other than practicing awareness of these body clues through body scanning.

Worksheet 4.1: Body Drawing

Identify specific parts of your body where you experience uncomfortable or upsetting body clues.

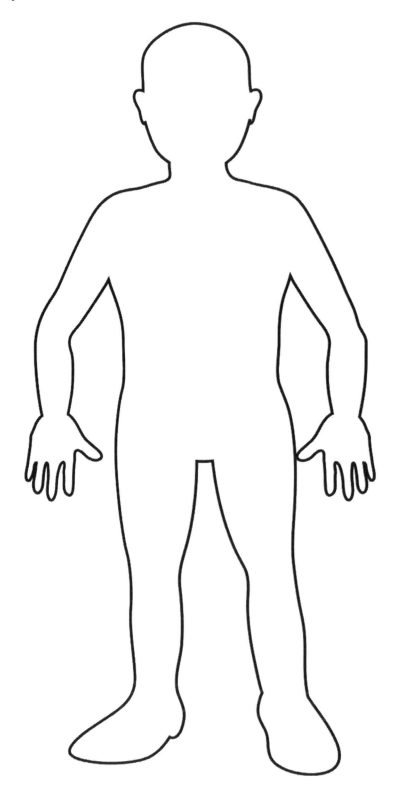

Worksheet 4.2: Monitoring How My Body Feels

Use this worksheet to keep track of the physical sensations you experience while doing sensational exposures. Note each exposure task you complete, as well as the physical sensations you experience (e.g., chest tightness, shortness of breath) and how strong they feel. Do you notice anything about your thoughts, emotions, or urges to use any emotional behaviors while doing these exposures?

Rating Scale:

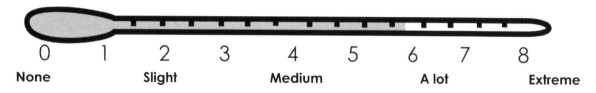

| 0 | 1 | 2 | 3 | 4 | 5 | 6 | 7 | 8 |
| None | | Slight | | Medium | | A lot | | Extreme |

Name of Sensational Exposure Task	Physical Sensations	Intensity of Sensation (0–8)	Notes (e.g. thoughts, emotions, desire to engage in emotional behaviors)

Form 4.1: Tracking the Before, During, and After

Each week, you will be asked to track the Before, During, and After of your emotional experiences. In order to change your emotional experiences, it is important that you understand the patterns that may occur (e.g., what triggers your emotional experiences, what happens as a result of your emotional experiences, etc.). This form will help you understand these patterns. By keeping this form and referring back to it later, you will start to see how changing one part of the pattern can change everything.

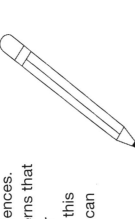

What happened Before? (What was the trigger?)	What happened During? (What was your emotional response to the trigger?)			What happened After? (What were the consequences of your emotional responses?)	
	Thoughts	Feelings	Behaviors	Short Term	Long Term

CHAPTER 5 | Being Flexible in Your Thinking

- To learn to be flexible in your thinking
- To learn about common thinking traps
- To use Detective Thinking to challenge your automatic thoughts
- To learn the steps of Problem Solving and begin to apply them to your own problems

Being Flexible in Your Thinking: Automatic and Alternative Interpretations

As you go through each day, you are constantly having thoughts and making decisions about the things going on around you, without even realizing it. If you get to school in the morning just as the bell begins to ring, for example, you might then run to your classroom right away. You know, without even thinking about it, that the bell means you are supposed to be in class. Or think about what happens when you or someone else is driving and the light turns red. You would probably put your foot on the brake to stop the car, without taking the time to think about what the red light means. We know how to act in these types of situations because they are so familiar to us that our brain takes shortcuts that allow us to act more quickly. What would happen if you had to stop and think about what a ringing school bell means, or about what a red traffic light means? You might end up being really late to class or running right through a stoplight! This process of interpreting a situation without thinking about it is called an **automatic interpretation**.

Our automatic interpretations are often helpful, like in the above examples, because they allow us to respond quickly to things in our environment. *However, sometimes our automatic interpretations may get us in trouble because they may not always be accurate or helpful.* There may be other, more accurate or more helpful interpretations that we miss because our brains are taking a shortcut. This is sometimes the case when we experience strong emotions. Our fear, sadness, anger, or other emotions may be affecting what kind of automatic interpretation we make in a situation. For example, when we feel sad or worried, we may tend to focus on the more negative parts of a situation. Focusing on the negative parts might then make us feel more sad and worried. When we feel happy or excited, we may have a more positive view of a situation, which would likely make us continue to feel good or even better than we did before. So, how we interpret these situations in our lives is really important, and learning to be flexible about our automatic interpretations might also be important!

Let's take an example. Imagine that you are talking with your teacher after class about how you did on a test. Your teacher praises you for doing a good job overall, but offers suggestions for improving so that you can do even better the next time. As you leave, your **automatic interpretation** might be that you didn't do well and the teacher was just being nice. If you continue to focus on the idea that the teacher was criticizing you or just giving you false praise, you would probably feel even worse. It might even lead to emotional behaviors in the future if you then avoid taking tests or spend too much time preparing because you think you're no good at test taking. However, your automatic interpretation is not the only way to think about your teacher's feedback. Instead, you might think that your test performance had strengths and weaknesses. This is called an **alternative interpretation**, or an interpretation that takes a different, more balanced or more realistic view. If you focus on this more neutral interpretation, you might use the situation as an opportunity to improve how you do on tests. You might also choose to focus on your teacher's praise in this situation, which would probably make you feel good. Not only do our emotions impact our interpretations of a situation, but our interpretations also impact our emotions.

Try to start paying attention to the thoughts that pop into your head during the day, especially in situations that make you feel strong emotions.

When you catch yourself making an automatic interpretation, consider if there are other, alternative thoughts that may also be accurate or may even be more accurate. Practicing this will help you to start being more flexible in the way you think about situations.

Thinking Traps

Sometimes a negative view of a given situation makes sense, but often a different interpretation, one that is more neutral or even positive, is much more realistic and helpful. However, some teens can get stuck on the same interpretation again and again and have a hard time seeing things a different way. Evaluating similar situations in the same way again and again despite facts and experiences suggesting that they may be different is called a **thinking trap** because it can be easy to get trapped in that way of thinking. Take a look at Worksheet 5.1: *Common Thinking Traps* at the end of this chapter. On those pages, you will see a list of the most common thinking traps that some teens tend to get stuck in, as well as an example of a thought that falls into each thinking trap. You may find that one or two of these thinking traps are much more common for you than the others.

Let's look at examples of some of the most common thinking traps. **Thinking the Worst** refers to the tendency to think that the worst possible outcome is going to happen. For example, if you text your friend and she doesn't text you back, you might be thinking the worst if you start thinking that she dislikes you and no longer wants to be friends. Or, you might be thinking the worst if you worry that if you don't wash your hands in a certain way, you might get a terrible disease. In both of these situations, you are thinking the worst because you believe that the outcome would be catastrophic, even though not getting a text back from your friend or not washing your hands in a certain way does not usually lead to terrible outcomes. Many people who get stuck in thinking the worst also believe that if that bad thing were to occur, they would not be able to deal with it or *cope* with it.

Jumping to Conclusions refers to thinking that the chances of something bad happening are much greater than they actually are. For example, if you see a storm coming, you might be jumping to conclusions if you start thinking that there is a very high chance of your house getting hit by lightning. When you realize that you are jumping to conclusions, it can sometimes be helpful and even surprising to look up information about the actual chance of your feared outcome occurring.

Let's look at one more example. **Ignoring the Positive** is another common thinking trap that refers to the tendency to only focus on the negative parts of a situation, without thinking of the positive aspects. Remember the test example we were discussing earlier? If you were ignoring the positive, you would only be focusing on your teacher's suggestions for improvement and ignoring the praise she gave you about the presentation.

HOME LEARNING ASSIGNMENT

Over the next week, try to catch yourself if you are falling into some of the thinking traps discussed in Worksheet 5.1: *Common Thinking Traps*. When you do catch yourself, write the thought you had in the lines underneath the thinking trap that the thought belongs to. At the end of the week, take a look at what you've written down. Do you notice that you are falling into some thinking traps more than others?

Your therapist may also ask you to continue to track your emotional experiences this week using Form 5.2: *Tracking the Before, During, and After*. This form can be found at the end of this chapter.

Using Detective Thinking to Challenge Your Automatic Interpretations

Now that you gotten some practice with identifying your automatic interpretations and deciding whether they fall into any thinking traps, let's talk about how to get yourself out of these thinking traps. It can be helpful to think of an automatic interpretation as one hypothesis or guess about what might be true in a given situation. In order to determine whether there is any support for this hypothesis, it is important to gather evidence and then to decide whether that evidence supports your hypothesis. In this treatment, you will be learning to treat your automatic interpretations as hypotheses that need to be evaluated.

We call the process of re-evaluating your automatic interpretations **Detective Thinking** because we want you to think about your interpretations or hypotheses the way a detective might—as something worth investigating. When we investigate our automatic interpretations, we are looking to see if there is any evidence to support, get rid of, or change our original interpretation. **Detective questioning** is one way of looking for evidence that involves asking ourselves questions to evaluate the evidence for our thoughts. If you turn to Worksheet 5.2: *Evaluating My Thoughts Using Detective Questioning*, you will see a list of example detective questions for three of the most common thinking traps. If you look at the questions carefully, you will notice that many of them are asking you to consider (1) why you are so certain that your feared outcome is true; (2) what else might be true based on your experiences; and (3) how bad it would actually be if your feared outcome did come true. Many of these questions can easily be applied to other thinking traps, and you will likely be able to think of other questions on your own as you are gathering evidence.

Take one of the automatic thoughts that you noted on Worksheet 5.1: *Common Thinking Traps*, and go through some of the detective questions to evaluate the evidence for that thought. Once you've done some detective questioning, do you feel as certain as you did before that your automatic interpretation is true?

Using detective questioning is just one step of Detective Thinking, but it's one of the most important ones! Now that you are starting to get the hang of detective questioning, let's learn about the other steps and put it all together.

Step 1. *Identify your automatic interpretation.* Just like you have already practiced, in this step you are identifying the automatic interpretation that is causing you to feel the strong emotion. Example: "If I don't get straight A's on my report card, I'll never get into a good college."

Step 2. *Identify whether you are falling into any thinking traps, and try to identify which one or ones.* Example: Thinking the Worst.

Step 3. *Evaluate the evidence for your automatic thought by using detective questioning (Worksheet 5.2), just as you have already practiced.*

Step 4. *After looking at your evidence, identify the most realistic or likely outcome.*

Step 5. *If the outcome from step 4 were to occur, could you deal or cope with it?* Sometimes, the realistic outcome you come up with in step 4 isn't fun, might bring up strong emotions, or isn't the way you would like the situation to turn out. However, is it the worst thing that could ever happen? Would you be able to get through it? How?

Now that you know the steps of Detective Thinking, you can start to practice using the steps with your own automatic interpretations, using

Worksheet 5.3: *Being a Detective—Steps for Detective Thinking*. Often, the best time to use Detective Thinking is *before* you find yourself in a situation that makes you feel strong emotions. This is because when you are in the middle of a situation that is making you sad or angry or nervous, you often feel so overwhelmed by the emotions that it is difficult for you to think flexibly about what else might be true. Therefore, if you can think ahead to things that may make you feel strong emotions in the future (e.g., if you know that large parties make you feel very nervous or having to look after your siblings makes you feel frustrated), you can do Detective Thinking ahead of time on the automatic interpretations you may have in response to those triggers.

Just because it is often best to use Detective Thinking before an emotional situation, however, this is not the only time you can use it! You can also use Detective Thinking if you notice that you are thinking about something that already happened in a way that is unhelpful or unrealistic, or if you notice that you are thinking over and over about something in the past.

HOME LEARNING ASSIGNMENT

Over the next week, try to think ahead to one or two situations in which you are likely to experience a strong emotion. Use Form 5.1: *Detective Thinking* to track your automatic interpretation, thinking trap(s), detective questions used to evaluate the evidence (e.g., What's happened in the past? What's the worst that could happen?), and your alternative or more realistic thought. Notice that the first row on this form has been filled in for you with an example. Your therapist may ask you to continue using this form to track your efforts at Detective Thinking over the next couple of sessions.

Your therapist may also ask you to continue to track your emotional experiences this week using Form 5.2: *Tracking the Before, During, and After*. This form can be found at the end of this chapter.

Getting Unstuck: Problem Solving

We all face problems every day, some small and some big. If you run out of milk for your cereal in the morning, you may have the problem of finding something else to eat for breakfast. An example of a bigger problem might be that you told your friend you would go see a movie with her on Sunday and don't want to disappoint her, but you remember that you have a big test you need to study for the next day. When problems come up—especially ones that make you feel angry, sad, worried, or other emotions—you may get stuck on one way of solving the problem. So far in this chapter, you have been practicing using Detective Thinking during times when you get stuck on one interpretation or way of thinking about a situation. **Problem Solving** is another skill that can help you get unstuck, and problem solving is for helping you think flexibly about other things that you can *do* about a situation.

Just like with Detective Thinking, Problem Solving has five very important steps. Let's go through each of them one by one. Your therapist may use Figure 5.1: *Getting Unstuck—Step-by-Step Example of Solving a Problem* to walk through this first example of problem solving with you.

Step 1. *Define the problem.* State the problem as clearly and as simply as possible. This step is really important because how you define the problem will influence what solutions you come up with.

Step 2. *Identify some solutions.* Try to come up with a number of possible solutions. The key to this step is not to evaluate them yet or decide whether they are good or bad. Just come up with as many solutions as possible, even if you think they might not work.

Step 3. *List the good things and bad things about each solution.* Try to come up with at least one good thing and one bad thing about each of the possible solutions from step 2.

Step 4. *Pick a solution and try it out.* Based on the good and bad things about each solution, pick one and try it out. Be specific about when and how you will put the solution into action.

Step 5. *If necessary, go through the process again.* Often, our first solution to a problem doesn't end up working out the way we'd like it to, or maybe doesn't end up working out at all. It's important to remember that this happens to everyone, and that this is okay. When this happens, you can either try one of the other solutions you already came up with, or you can go back to step 1 and try again. Trying the first time and not succeeding may help you to change the way you define the problem or think of other solutions.

When trying to figure out how to solve a problem there is a set of steps we can use every time. In fact, these may be steps that you are sometimes using without even realizing it.

The first step is simple, **Define the Problem**. Be careful; the way you define the problem will influence the solutions you arrive at. Try to keep the problem as simple as possible.

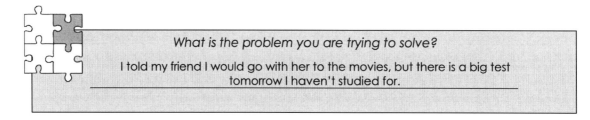

What is the problem you are trying to solve?

I told my friend I would go with her to the movies, but there is a big test tomorrow I haven't studied for.

Now, try to determine all the possible solutions or all the things you could do to solve the problem. Remember not to judge your options right now, just list out as many options as you can.

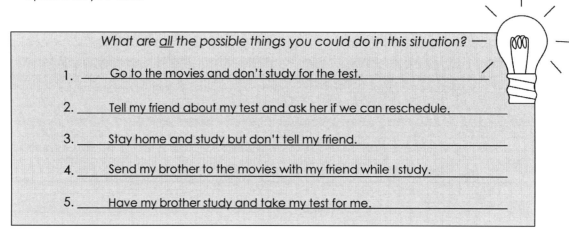

What are all the possible things you could do in this situation?

1.   Go to the movies and don't study for the test.

2.   Tell my friend about my test and ask her if we can reschedule.

3.   Stay home and study but don't tell my friend.

4.   Send my brother to the movies with my friend while I study.

5.   Have my brother study and take my test for me.

Now that you've listed out some possible solutions, let's start to think about what is good and what is bad about each of the options. What are the likely outcomes of each solution?

Using the chart on the next page, write down the good and bad things about each of the solutions listed above in the appropriate column.

Figure 5.1

Getting Unstuck—Step-by-Step Example of Solving a Problem

	What are the **good** things about each solution?	What are the **bad** things about each solution? 
Solution 1.	I get to go to the movies and not disappoint my friend.	I might not do well on my test if I don't study.
Solution 2.	I might do better on my test if I study and still might get to go to the movies another time.	I might disappoint my friend, and maybe she can't reschedule.
Solution 3.	I might do better on my test if I study and don't have to worry about having to tell my friend.	My friend might get really mad if I don't call her and just don't show up to the movie.
Solution 4.	I might do better on my test if I study and my friend might not be disappointed.	My friend might not want to go to the movies with my brother and might be disappointed that I am not there.
Solution 5.	I get to go to the movies and do not disappoint my friend.	My teacher will notice that my brother is taking the test instead of me and I will get in trouble.

Now, circle the solution you think is the best one and try it out!

Pick a specific time that you plan to try out your solution:

I am going to try out telling my friend and will ask her if we can reschedule tomorrow.
_____

Figure 5.1
Continued

HOME LEARNING ASSIGNMENT

Over the next week, pay attention to the problems that come up for you. Choose at least one and go through the steps of Problem Solving using Worksheet 5.4: *Getting Unstuck—Steps for Solving a Problem*. You don't need to select a huge problem, but try to pick a problem that brings up some emotions for you. After going through the steps of Problem Solving, be sure to try your solution out and think about how it worked. Did you solve the problem? Do you need to go back to one of the other steps and try again?

Throughout this chapter, you should also continue to track your emotional experiences each week by completing Form 5.2: *Tracking the Before, During, and After*. If doing both the Detective Thinking or Problem Solving home learning and your Tracking the Before, During, and After forms feels like a lot more work than you can do in one week, please make sure to talk to your therapist about this so that he or she can tell you which form is more important for you to focus on.

Now that you have been tracking your emotional experiences for a number of weeks, do you notice any patterns? It might be helpful to discuss this with your therapist.

Worksheet 5.1: Common Thinking Traps

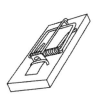 How we feel is directly related to what we believe and how we think. In any situation we can have different types of thoughts. While some thoughts can make us feel calm or happy, other thoughts can make us feel anxious, angry or down. We call these thoughts **thinking traps** because sometimes we get stuck in a pattern of unhelpful thinking.

Here is a list of common thinking traps. We cover some of these in session, and some may be new to you. Put a checkmark in the box next to each thinking trap that you sometimes fall into, and come up with your own example in the space provided.

☐ **Jumping to Conclusions** – Thinking that the chances of something bad happening are much greater than they actually are.

Example: You think that there is a 90% chance that your plane is going to crash (when the real chance is more like 0.000013%)

Your example:

_____

_____

☐ **Thinking the Worst** – Telling yourself that the very worst is happening or is going to happen, without thinking of other, less negative ways the situation could turn out.

Example: If your parents are late getting home, you assume that they have been in an accident.

Your example:

_____

_____

☐ **Ignoring the Positive** – Telling yourself that your achievements or successes "don't count" and that you just "got lucky." Always focusing on the negative rather than the positive.

Example: You tell yourself that you only made a good grade on a test because the questions just happened to be easy.

Your example:

_____

_____

☐ **Black-and-White Thinking** – Thinking that a situation has to be either one way or the other, with no possibilities in between.

Example: Believing that if you don't get 100% on a test you are a failure.

Your example:

_____

_____

☐ **Fortune Telling** – Predicting that something negative is going to happen in the future, as if you were gazing into a crystal ball.

Example: You decide not to perform in a recital because you are sure that you are going to mess up.

Your example:

_____

_____

☐ **Mind Reading** – Believing you know what others are thinking without considering other, more likely, possibilities. Making no effort to check out what others might truly be thinking.

Example: You think that a girl in your class definitely does not like you, even though you've never talked to her.

Your example:

_____

_____

☐ **Emotional Reasoning** – Thinking something must be true because you "feel" (actually believe) it so strongly, ignoring or disbelieving evidence to the contrary.

Example: If you feel it in your gut that your parents are in a car accident, you believe it is really true, even though they told you they might run a little late.

Your example:

_____

_____

☐ **Labeling** – Putting a fixed, global label on yourself or others without considering that the evidence might more reasonably lead to a less disastrous conclusion.

Example: Saying to yourself, "I am ugly," or "I am stupid."

Your example:

_____

_____

☐ **"Should" and "Must" Statements** – Having a precise, fixed idea of how you or others should behave, and overestimating how bad it is that these expectations are not met.

Example: Believing that if you and your classmates don't walk in a straight line like your teacher told you to, your teacher will call your parents and you will get in big trouble.

Your example:

_____

_____

☐ **Magical Thinking** – Believing that, through your actions, you have the power to control things that you actually can't control.

Example: Thinking that if you call your mom on her cell phone she won't get into an accident.

Your example:

_____

_____

Detective Questions are questions you can ask when evaluating any automatic interpretations or thoughts. Some examples are listed here. Most of these questions work well with many of the thinking traps, but you may need to experiment to see which ones work best for you. You may also be able to think of other detective questions that are not already on this list.

Am I Sure?

1. Am I 100% certain that _____will happen?

2. What evidence do I have for this fear or belief?

3. Do I have a crystal ball? How can I be sure that I know the answer?

4. Could there be any other explanations?

5. Am I missing out on other things that could happen because of my intense emotions?

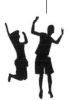

How Bad Would It Actually Be?

1. What is the worst that could happen? How bad is that?

2. If_____happened, could I cope with it? How would I handle it?

3. So what?

4. Have I been able to cope with_____in the past?

5. If_____happened, would anything good come out of it?

What Has Happened Before?

1. What happened in the past in this situation?

2. Based on my past experience with this situation, what has happened most often?

3. What has happened to other people in this situation?

Given your answers to these questions, what is an alternative way of looking at this situation?

Worksheet 5.3: Being a Detective—Steps for Detective Thinking

Detective Thinking is a tool you can use to help look for evidence and clues about your thoughts or interpretations to help you figure out if you are falling into one of the "thinking traps." Use this worksheet to help you walk through your Detective Thinking steps. Refer to the description of each step in the workbook for more instructions on how to do Detective Thinking.

The first step is to **Identify the Interpretation.** Try to get at the **emotional thought behind the interpretation**. For example, rather than, "If I don't get straight A's it will be terrible," the core interpretation may be, "If I don't get straight A's on my report card I'll never get into the colleges I really want to go to!"

What is your interpretation?

_____

Now, try to determine whether you are falling into any thinking traps (e.g., Jumping to Conclusions, Thinking the Worst, Ignoring the Positive). Refer to Worksheet 5.1: *Common Thinking Traps* for a description of several thinking traps.

What thinking traps are you falling into?

_____

_____

The next step is to evaluate the evidence using some of the detective questions listed on Worksheet 5.2: *Evaluating My Thoughts Using Detective Questioning.*

Detective Question	Answer
_____	_____
_____	_____
_____	_____

After evaluating the evidence, the next step is to **choose a realistic outcome.** Finally, consider whether you would be able to **cope with that outcome if it were to occur.**

Form 5.1: Detective Thinking

Automatic Interpretation (Thought)	Identify "Thinking Trap"	Strategy/Questions to evaluate evidence	Alternative Thought
The plane I am taking to vacation will crash.	Thinking the worst	Detective Questions. How likely is it? What has happened in the past?	It is very unlikely that the plane will crash.

Worksheet 5.4: Getting Unstuck—Steps for Solving a Problem

When trying to figure out how to solve a problem there is a set of steps we can use every time. In fact, these may be steps that you are sometimes using without even realizing it.

The first step is simple, **Define the Problem**. Be careful; the way you define the problem will influence the solutions you arrive at. Try to keep the problem as simple as possible.

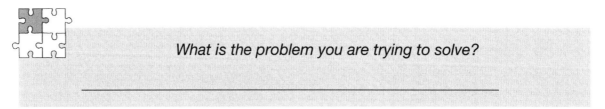

What is the problem you are trying to solve?

_____

Now, try to determine all the possible solutions or all the things you could do to solve the problem. Remember not to judge your options right now, just list out as many options as you can.

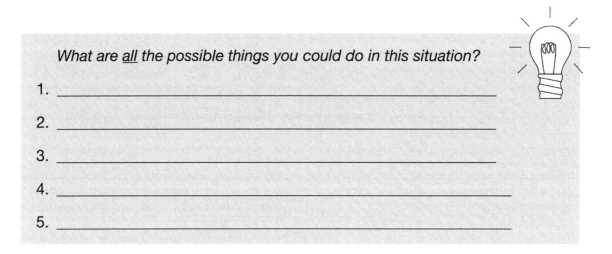

What are all the possible things you could do in this situation?

1. _____

2. _____

3. _____

4. _____

5. _____

Now that you've listed out some possible solutions, let's start to think about what is good and what is bad about each of the options. What are the likely outcomes of each solution?

Using the chart on the next page, write down the good and bad things about each of the solutions you listed above in the appropriate column.

	What are the **good** things about each solution?	What are the **bad** things about each solution?
Solution 1.		
Solution 2.		
Solution 3.		
Solution 4.		
Solution 5.		

Now, circle the solution you think is the best one and try it out!

Pick a specific time that you plan to try out your solution:

_____

If the solution you choose doesn't work, go through the process again. With the information you now have, re-evaluate your options and pick another solution to try.

Form 5.2: Tracking the Before, During, and After

Each week, you will be asked to track the Before, During, and After of your emotional experiences. In order to change your emotional experiences, it is important that you understand the patterns that may occur (e.g., what triggers your emotional experiences, what happens as a result of your emotional experiences, etc.). This form will help you understand these patterns. By keeping them and referring back to them later, you can see how changing one part of the pattern can change everything.

What happened **Before**? (What was the trigger?)	What happened **During**? (What was your emotional response to the trigger?)			What happened **After**? (What were the consequences of your emotional responses?)	
	Thoughts	**Feelings**	**Behaviors**	**Short Term**	**Long Term**

CHAPTER 6 — Awareness of Emotional Experiences

- To learn how to be aware of emotional experiences
- To learn the steps for practicing present-moment awareness
- To learn how to use nonjudgmental awareness to be more accepting of emotional experiences
- To apply present-moment and nonjudgmental awareness to emotional experiences

Increasing Awareness of our Emotional Experiences

Think of a time when you were so caught up in your thoughts or emotions that you were not even aware of what you were doing or how you ended up doing it. Maybe you were so caught up thinking about your parent telling you that you couldn't go to a party that you didn't even talk to your friends during lunch, and as the day went on, you felt yourself becoming more worried, sad, or angry. Or maybe you were so worried about how you would perform in a basketball practice that you couldn't stop thinking about it all day. Finally, you decided you would just rather stay home and not go to basketball after all. Sometimes things like this happen because our strong emotions can stop us from noticing, enjoying, or appreciating what is happening in the present moment, which makes us more likely to engage in emotional behaviors. When people try to refocus on what is going on in the present moment, sometimes they realize that their emotional thoughts have gotten them much more upset than the trigger that started bothering them in the first place!

Not focusing on the present moment is sometimes referred to as being on automatic pilot, or **autopilot** for short. When a plane or subway train is on autopilot, it is set to run itself for a little while. When we talk about you being on autopilot, though, we are referring to times when you are doing things throughout the day without really thinking about what you are doing. For example, many of us can complete our morning routines (e.g., showering, getting dressed, brushing our teeth) without really focusing on each step of the process. When you are on autopilot in this way, you are not as focused on the details of what is going on around you. We are suggesting that you try to minimize the time you are on autopilot and instead try to stay in the "here and now." This concept might sound weird to you—because you may feel like you are TOO aware of your thoughts and experiences during situations that cause you to experience strong emotions since these emotions are bothering you so much! But, in reality, we may just be focusing too much on unhelpful ideas about ourselves, past events, or worries about the future during these times—not the present moment! As a result, being on autopilot can keep us stuck in a very strong emotion twister and lead us to engage in unhelpful emotional behaviors.

Present-moment awareness can help us get out of autopilot mode by slowing down our thoughts and helping us become more aware of what is really going on within and around us. When we are practicing present-moment awareness, we are focusing on one thing at a time and fully participating in the "here and now," not focusing on the future (which hasn't happened yet) or the past (which we can't change).

Learning the Steps for Practicing Present-Moment Awareness

There are three steps to follow when practicing present-moment awareness:

1. **Notice it** (wordlessly notice your environment and emotional experiences).
2. **Say something about it** (label the details of your experience out loud or just to yourself).
3. **Experience it** (use all of your senses to fully experience the moment without distractions).

In order to *notice* the present moment, you should try to be aware of what you see, hear, smell, taste, or touch. To *say something about it*, try to use words to label and describe your experience to yourself in your mind (or out loud to your therapist or another supportive person). It is important to not try to make decisions about what each of your thoughts or experiences mean, but rather just notice what is happening in the present, much like the play-by-play commentary used in sports. Label what you see, smell, taste, touch, and hear. For example, if you are drawing or coloring, describe the details of what you are doing. What shapes are you drawing? How much force are you using to color? Does the crayon have a smell? Does the crayon feel cold between your fingers? Are there textures that you notice or feel? What colors do you observe? What are your thoughts about what you are doing?

To *experience it*, let yourself fully be involved in the present moment. What does this mean exactly? Mostly, it's being as engaged as you can be in the here and now and using your senses of sight, smell, touch, taste, and hearing to be in the moment as much as you can. Let yourself experience the moment fully with all of your attention and with as few distractions as possible. For example, when going for a walk, fully experience the present moment by noticing the breeze as you walk, the trees you are passing by, the way the sunlight feels on your skin, the movements your legs make, and what it feels like when your feet push against the ground. It's certainly okay if you get distracted! Just notice that you became distracted and bring yourself back to the present moment.

You can start practicing present-moment awareness by bringing your awareness to everyday objects and experiences. For example, you can begin by noticing your breath as you inhale and exhale as well as the body movements and sensations that occur with each breath. Other examples of bringing present-moment awareness to everyday situations include being fully aware of the experiences of walking or eating, sitting at your desk, completing chores, or being outdoors. Practicing awareness of the present moment like this will help increase your enjoyment of the things you are doing in the here and now, and it will also keep you from getting stuck in distracting or upsetting worry thoughts about the past or future.

After practicing present-moment awareness with everyday objects or routine situations, you can begin to bring this awareness to your own emotional experiences. You can start by bringing your awareness to your bodily sensations during strong emotions by using **body scanning**, much like you did in Chapter 4. You can then begin to notice and label your thoughts as they go through your mind. Then bring your awareness to your emotional behaviors (see Worksheet 6.1: *Notice it, Say Something About It, Experience It*).

Bringing Acceptance to Our Awareness of Emotional Experiences

Nonjudgmental awareness is a form of present-moment awareness. It is all about having a compassionate, kind, and accepting way of thinking about what is going on inside and around us. In nonjudgmental awareness, you are being encouraged to approach your emotional experience—whatever that may be—with kindness and understanding, much like we would treat a friend! For example, you may call yourself dumb for getting some questions wrong on your math homework or call yourself a failure for making a mistake while playing the guitar, but would you call your close friend dumb or a failure if those things happened to him? Chances are you would be more accepting, understanding, or even compassionate if these things happened to your friend. This is the type of nonjudgmental awareness to practice bringing to your own emotional experiences.

Being nonjudgmentally aware of our emotional experiences can help us change our emotional behaviors. For example, in the above situation, you might be more likely to try again and allow yourself to perform better in school or on the guitar if you adopt a nonjudgmental attitude about such small setbacks, while judging yourself might result in emotional behaviors such as procrastinating doing your homework in fear of getting more problems wrong or skipping guitar practice.

After practicing present-moment awareness a few times, you can begin to bring nonjudgmental awareness into your awareness practice of everyday objects and situations as well as your own emotional experience. The first step in practicing nonjudgmental awareness is simply *noticing* when you are labeling an object, thought, person, or situation as good or bad. After you notice that you are making that type of judgment, try to *replace it* with a more neutral or factual description. For example, rather than describing a food as "gross," try to focus on its flavors and what it feels like in your mouth. Instead of describing a tree along your walk as "ugly," notice and tell yourself about its colors, texture, and the height of its branches. And instead of labeling a thought as "bad," try to just describe the thought you are having in as much detail as possible. You can even challenge yourself to practice nonjudgmental awareness by noticing and telling yourself about things you actually have very strong feelings about, while trying to use language that is as neutral as possible and stick to the facts.

Applying Present-Moment and Nonjudgmental Awareness to Our Strong Emotions

Once you get the hang of being aware of experiences inside your body and around it using present-moment and nonjudgmental awareness, you can begin to practice these skills together by using them at times when you feel strong emotions. You may choose to practice by listening to music or watching a video clip, reading or writing a story, or engaging in some other activity that causes a strong emotion. Your therapist will work with you in session to identify which exercises are best for you and help you practice this idea together.

While engaging in these practices, your job is to pay attention to both the emotions you experience and the parts of your emotional experiences, including the thoughts, physical sensations, and behaviors that are associated with these emotions. Use your present-moment awareness skills to notice and tell yourself about the different parts of your emotions, and experience these fully by focusing on these as much as you can, rather than distracting yourself or pushing your thoughts or sensations away. If you notice any judgments about your experience, try to restate those judgments using more neutral or kind language that just sticks to the facts.

One thing you might do with your therapist is write a brief story about a situation in your life when you experienced a strong emotion. As you write this story and read it back to yourself and/or your therapist, you can use your present-moment and nonjudgmental awareness skills to pay attention to the emotions, thoughts, and physical sensations you experience without judging them or trying to push them away. If you and your therapist decide to do this activity, you may use Worksheet 6.2: *Emotion Story*.

HOME LEARNING ASSIGNMENT

Over the next week, you will practice present-moment and nonjudgmental awareness. Use Form 6.1: *Awareness Practice Monitoring* to track your practice. Nonjudgmental and present-moment awareness can feel different, unrealistic, or hard to do, but it's not something you have to do perfectly in order for it to be helpful. Like any other skill, it takes practice. Try practicing daily. Five minutes is all it takes!

You can also continue to track the Before, During, and After of additional emotional experiences throughout the week using Form 6.2: *Tracking the Before, During, and After.*

If doing both *Awareness Practice Monitoring* and *Tracking the Before, During, and After* forms feels like a lot more work than you can do in one week, please make sure to talk to your therapist about this so that he or she can tell you which form is more important for you to focus on right now.

Worksheet 6.1: Notice It, Say Something About It, Experience It

Noticing it, saying something about it, and experiencing it can help you practice present-moment awareness.

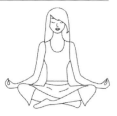

Notice it:

What did you notice? Name the object, food, location, person, event, or emotion that you observed using present-moment awareness:

_____

_____

Say something about it:

Describe what you noticed in as much detail as you can (e.g., what colors, textures, tastes, temperatures, sensations, smells, and/or people do you notice?). Remember not to make any judgments or interpretations, just describe what is there:

_____

_____

_____

_____

_____

Experience it:

How are you staying in the present moment?

_____

_____

Remember: When you notice a distracting thought or judgment, gently bring yourself back to the present moment.

Form 6.1: Awareness Practice Monitoring

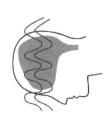

Present-moment awareness (PMA) and nonjudgmental awareness (NJA) are skills you can practice on your own. Use this form to chart your present-moment and/or nonjudgmental awareness practice for the week. First, identify the feeling you are having and rate its intensity using the 0–8 scale. After you complete the awareness activity, rate your mood again and write down any comments you have about the activity.

Date	What emotion(s) are you feeling?	Rating BEFORE (0–8)	Practiced PMA or NJA?	Rating AFTER (0–8)	Thoughts, comments, or obstacles
			YES NO		
			YES NO		
			YES NO		
			YES NO		
			YES NO		
			YES NO		
			YES NO		
			YES NO		

Extreme — 8
A lot — 7, 6
Medium — 5, 4, 3
Some — 2, 1
None — 0

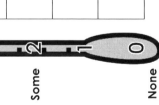

Worksheet 6.2: Emotion Story

Write a brief story about a situation that happened to you in which you felt a strong emotion. It should be personal and about <u>your</u> life, if possible, but if not – it's okay to tell the story of someone else you know. Wherever possible, use "I statements" and "feeling words" to describe what happened. You may feel strong emotions while writing this, but that's okay. We will use this assignment to help with being aware of the emotions that such a story brings up for you.

_____

_____

_____

_____

_____

_____

_____

_____

_____

_____

_____

_____

_____

_____

What kinds of emotions were you aware of while writing this story? Please list these below:

Did you have any negative reactions to these feelings, such as distracting yourself, avoiding, or otherwise trying to get away from your feelings? If so, please note these below:

Form 6.2: Tracking the Before, During, and After

Each week, you will be asked to track the Before, During, and After of your emotional experiences. In order to change your emotional experiences, it is important that you understand the patterns that may occur (e.g., what triggers your emotional experiences, what happens as a result of your emotional experiences, etc.). This form will help you understand these patterns. By keeping them and referring back to them later, you can see how changing one part of the pattern can change everything.

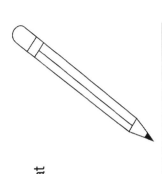

What happened <u>Before?</u> (What was the trigger?)	What happened <u>During?</u> (What was your emotional response to the trigger?)			What happened <u>After?</u> (What were the consequences of your emotional responses?)	
	Thoughts	Feelings	Behaviors	Short Term	Long Term

CHAPTER 7 Situational Emotion Exposures

GOALS

- To review the skills you have learned so far in this treatment
- To create Form 7.1: *Emotional Behavior Form* to help you decide which emotional behaviors to focus on next in treatment
- To learn what to expect when you begin situational emotion exposures
- To create an emotion ladder for breaking down situations that bring up strong emotions

Reviewing Your Skills

In this treatment so far, you have spent a lot of time learning about the different emotions you experience and about the things your emotions make you feel, think, and do. By now, you are probably an expert on noticing your emotional experiences. You probably also have a very good understanding of what your emotions want you to *do* (emotional behaviors). For many teens, becoming more aware of their emotional behaviors is enough to make them begin to think about acting opposite to what the emotional behavior is telling them to do. In Chapter 3 of this treatment, you started to practice acting opposite to your emotional behaviors by participating in a behavioral experiment. You learned how doing activities that are enjoyable, even when you don't feel like it, can help improve your mood. In this chapter, we will be continuing to practice acting opposite to what our emotional behaviors are telling us to do by *approaching* instead of *avoiding* situations that make us feel very sad, afraid, worried, or frustrated. This new type of experiment is called a **situational emotion exposure**, and we will explain what that phrase means on the next few pages.

For now, let's think back on all the skills you have learned so far. As you review these skills, think about which ones have been most useful for you.

1. **Identifying Your Emotions:** In Chapter 1, you learned that emotions are normal, natural, and necessary. Emotions are not bad or dangerous, although it might feel like they can be. We have emotions for a reason, and experiencing emotions is part of being human, so maybe getting rid of them isn't the answer. By now, you can probably identify the emotions you're experiencing, including the three parts of an emotional experience AND the Before, During, and After associated with the emotion. This understanding can come in handy, so let's not forget about it.

2. **Acting Opposite:** In Chapter 3, you were introduced to the concept of "acting opposite," which means noticing what your emotional behavior is telling you to do and doing something different. You learned about opposite actions for different emotions and then practiced a behavioral experiment where you acted opposite to feelings of sadness by purposely choosing to do enjoyable activities even when you didn't feel like it. Behavioral experiments like this are important because they show us that changing the way we act in a situation, so that we are no longer using an emotional behavior, can actually change our emotional experience. In Chapter 4, you practiced acting opposite again by participating in activities that brought up strong body sensations without doing anything to reduce the strength of those sensations.

3. **Identifying Your Automatic Interpretations:** The human brain naturally focuses on certain aspects of a situation and gives meaning to those aspects. This allows you to quickly interpret the world around you, which allows you to quickly respond to the situation. This process of interpreting a given situation without thinking about it is called an automatic interpretation. Your automatic interpretations may or may not be accurate. In fact, there are often several possible interpretations (or ways to think about) any given situation. If your automatic interpretations are not accurate or helpful, you can re-evaluate them to see if anything else might be true.

4. **Detective Thinking:** Once you are able to identify your interpretations and evaluate whether you are falling into any thinking traps,

the next step is to learn the skills needed to get yourself out of these thinking traps. This includes gathering some evidence to evaluate the interpretations you make to figure out if they are realistic. Detective Thinking is a skill you can use to help you do this.

5. **Problem Solving**: Just as you can get stuck in thinking traps, you can also feel stuck in the choices you make. Use the Problem Solving steps to help you figure out what your options are and whether the option you are choosing is really the one you want to use.

6. **Present-Moment Awareness:** Present-moment awareness means fully participating in the "here and now," not in the future (which hasn't happened yet) or in the past (which we can't change). Practice present-moment awareness by noticing things around and inside of you using all of your senses, saying something about these observations, and allowing yourself to experience the "here and now."

7. **Nonjudgmental Awareness:** Nonjudgmental awareness, one type of present-moment awareness, is a kind and accepting awareness of what is going on inside and around us. We do not want to judge our experiences as right, wrong, good, or bad, but rather approach our experiences with empathy and understanding, much like we would toward a friend.

Now that you have these skills in your toolbox, you can use them whenever you need them. If you feel confused about any of these skills or feel like you are not using them, now might be a good time to review these skills in more detail by rereading some of the previous chapters and by talking with your therapist about when and how to use them. Your therapist will also help guide you in using some of these skills during the exposures that you will begin in this chapter.

Your Emotional Behavior Form

With your therapist, you will now create what we call an **Emotional Behavior Form** (Form 7.1). By now, you probably have a pretty good idea of the situations that make you feel strong emotions and things that you do as a result of feeling these emotions. As you create this list with your therapist, you may realize that a lot of the emotional behaviors that you were doing at the beginning of treatment have been replaced with more helpful behaviors. That's great! It's also okay if there are a number of emotional behaviors you still need to work on. Some teens have items on their list that focus on one emotion, like anxiety, while other teens have items on their list that focus on a range of different emotions. You should work with your therapist to make sure that this list includes things and situations that bring up all the emotions that make you feel uncomfortable, and the things you do when you feel those uncomfortable emotions. This list may not feel like the most fun thing to create, because it may remind you that there is still work to be done! But this form can be very useful at this moment to help you and your therapist know which kinds of situational emotion exposures to work on going forward.

As you create Form 7.1: *Emotional Behavior Form* with your therapist, it may be helpful to keep the following in mind:

- **Be specific**. Just like when you were making your SMART goals in Chapter 1, it is important to be specific about the situations that make you feel frustrated, nervous, or sad. For example, "Going to the counselor to avoid running in gym class" is much more specific than "Avoiding gym class."
- **Focus on the behavior**. Because behavioral experiments are all about changing what you *do* in situations that make you feel strong emotions, try to be specific about the behaviors you use. For example, "Washing my hands when I feel worried about germs" is much better than "Worrying about germs."
- **Think about what *you* want to work on.** Your goals for treatment may differ from what your parents or friends think you should work on. As you create your Emotional Behavior Form, try to think about what feels important to you and the situations that bother you the most.

You may wish to begin by using a blank piece of paper or scratch paper to brainstorm situations or objects that trigger strong emotions, as well as the emotional behaviors you typically use in response to those triggers. Once you have come up with some different items, you can then rate the intensity of the emotions you experience for each one. Write each item down on your Emotional Behavior Form in order of emotional intensity, placing the one with the lowest emotion rating at the bottom and the one with the highest emotion rating at the top. For some teens, it is helpful to see an example of a completed Emotional Behavior Form. We have provided one in Figure 7.1, in case you would like to take a look at examples of emotional behaviors that teens might put on their list.

Use this form to identify and describe situations that cause you to feel strong emotions, as well as the emotional behaviors you use in these situations. Using the Emotions Scale thermometer below, rate how much uncomfortable *emotion* you experience in each situation. When creating this list, think of behaviors like avoidance, escape or other undesired actions (like aggression) which you may wish to change during treatment. As time goes on in treatment, you can use the last column (Did you work on this?) to see how much progress you've made on these behaviors over time.

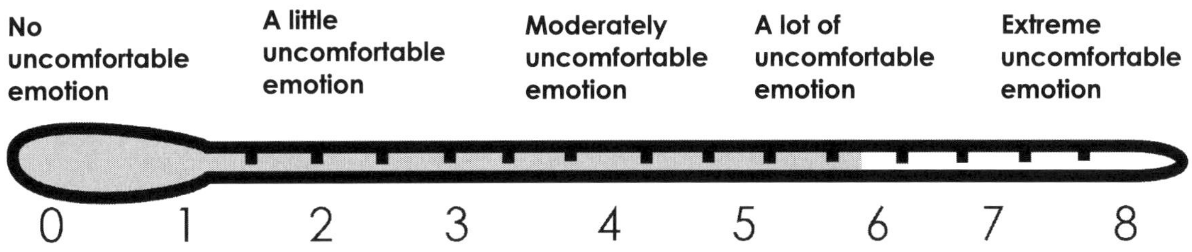

No uncomfortable emotion	**A little uncomfortable emotion**	**Moderately uncomfortable emotion**	**A lot of uncomfortable emotion**	**Extreme uncomfortable emotion**

0   1   2   3   4   5   6   7   8

Situation	Emotional Behavior	Emotion 0-8	Did you work on it? (Y/N)
Making presentations	Avoidance	7	
Having lunch at school	Sitting alone to avoid people	6	
Calling someone I don't know well to ask them to hang out	Avoidance	6	
My grandparents coming over to visit	Avoidance, Staying in my room	5	
Feeling frustrated about Algebra homework	Procrastination	4	
Going to the park (might see a snake)	Staying off the grass	4	
Disagreeing with my friends about something	Not expressing my opinion	3	
Walking to first period class	Taking the long way so nobody can talk to me	3	
Having to talk to store clerks and waiters	Not making eye contact	3	
Movies or tv shows with break-up scenes	Avoidance, Looking Away	2	

Figure 7.1

Sample Completed Emotional Behavior Form

Situational Emotion Exposures

In this part of treatment, you will be putting all of your skills to use as you begin to enter or experience situations you may have been avoiding because they bring up emotions. This is called a **situational emotion exposure**. When you began this treatment, you might have wondered why you would *want* to purposely do things to make yourself feel strong emotions like anxiety, sadness, or anger. After all, isn't the problem that you experience *too much* of these emotions? By now, you are probably beginning to realize that pushing your emotions away or avoiding situations that make you feel strong emotions may feel good in the short term, but these strategies don't get rid of the emotion in the long term, and they often create other problems. Let's take a look at why this happens.

Figure 7.2: *Emotion Curve: Avoidance/Escape* shows an emotion that starts low and then quickly grows. You might experience something like this if you are very afraid of dogs, and you are walking down the street when a dog suddenly begins to approach you. The black vertical line shows the point at

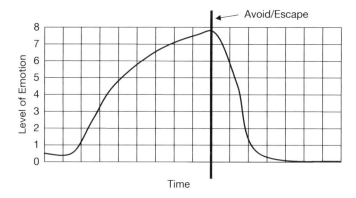

Figure 7.2

Emotion Curve: Avoidance/Escape

which you choose to get away from the thing that is triggering your emotional experience, like turning around and running in the opposite direction of the dog. Notice that when you escape the situation, the level of your emotion quickly goes down. Seems like a good idea, right? If you recall the **cycle of avoidance** from Chapter 2, you will remember that avoidance is not usually a strategy that works very well for managing your emotions.

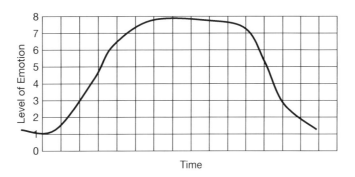

Figure 7.3

Emotion Curve: Habituation

Let's look at the next graph (Figure 7.3: *Emotion Curve: Habituation*) to see what might happen if you didn't avoid or escape the dog or other things that trigger uncomfortable emotions. Figure 7.3 shows what will often happen if you do not avoid or escape the trigger or situation that is making you feel a strong emotion. Although your emotion doesn't go down as quickly, you will notice that it still decreases and becomes less intense over time. By allowing your uncomfortable emotions to just be there, without trying to get away from the thing triggering the emotional experience or do something to lessen the emotional experience, your uncomfortable emotion will gradually become less intense. This is called **habituation**.

You should know that your strong emotion may not completely go away or return to "0" the first time. Some teens may not even notice much decrease in their emotion the first time they do an exposure, and they may need to repeat the exposure several times before they begin to feel better. Let's see what happens as you practice staying in the situation or sticking with the emotion over time.

As Figure 7.4: *Emotion Curve: Habituation with Practice* illustrates, the more you practice staying in the situation or sticking with the emotion, the more your emotion tends to become less intense and last for a shorter period of time. To return to the dog example, the more you stay around dogs without trying to escape or avoid them, the more your fear lessens over time.

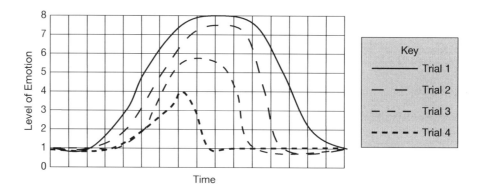

Figure 7.4

Emotion Curve: Habituation with Practice

While your uncomfortable body sensations may decrease during exposures, this is not the only (or even the most important) thing that happens
during situational emotion exposures! You also learn that the bad outcome you thought was going to occur often doesn't happen, or it's much
less dangerous or upsetting than you thought it was going to be. Then,
the next time you are in the same or a similar situation, you might remind
yourself of the new lessons and experiences you have had in such situations. In addition to gaining new knowledge about what is most likely
to happen in a situation, you also become more confident in your ability
to get through even very uncomfortable emotions without doing anything to get rid of them. As your confidence grows, the emotion begins to
bother you less and less with time.

Most exposure practices we have discussed so far involve just approaching (versus staying away from, or avoiding) some situation or thing.
There are also times your therapist may ask you to do an exposure
with what we call **response prevention**, which adds a small twist to
this process. Response prevention is really helpful when we find that
we are engaging in emotional behaviors (like washing our hands over
and over) because of an emotional thought that won't seem to go away
very easily (like the idea that you have something dirty on your hands,
as in the handwashing example). In response prevention, your therapist may ask you to be aware of that emotional thought while keeping
yourself from doing the emotional behavior. As you keep away from
doing that emotional behavior, you may feel less distressed as time
passes or with continued practice, similar to the way typical emotion
exposures work!

As you begin to do exposures, you will likely experience something similar to the patterns illustrated in these emotion graphs. The first time you allow yourself to experience situations or emotions you have been avoiding, with the help of your therapist, you may experience strong emotions and may want to act on your emotional behaviors. You should know that this is completely normal and okay! Try to use your present-moment and nonjudgmental awareness skills and experience the emotion without doing anything to get rid of it. Pay attention to any **safety behaviors** you may want to use, like distracting yourself from the emotion or situation, only entering the situation if you have someone with you, or carrying something that makes you feel better, like medicine or water. Using these safety behaviors can prevent you from fully experiencing your emotions or can make you feel like you are only okay because you used the safety behavior.

Creating an Emotion Ladder for Your Situational Emotion Exposures

As you begin to do situational emotion exposures, you and your therapist may take some ideas about situations or things that exposure would be helpful for from your Emotional Behavior Form and break them down into smaller, achievable steps. For example, if one of your emotional behaviors is "Avoiding giving speeches in front on my class," it might feel too difficult at first to immediately stand up and give a speech, and you might not always have the opportunity to do something like this even if you did feel ready. For items like this, it may be helpful to break them down into a series of smaller steps so that you can gradually work up to the emotional behavior on your list. In the case of giving a speech, some smaller steps might be:

1. Giving a short, 2-minute prepared speech in front of my parents
2. Giving a short, 2-minute prepared speech in front of my entire family over the weekend
3. Giving a short, 2-minute prepared speech in front of my two best friends
4. Giving a short, 2-minute speech in front of my younger brother's friends
5. Presenting my speech in front of the class

Use Form 7.3: *My Emotion Ladder* to break down the next item on your Emotional Behavior Form into at least three or four specific, achievable steps. Write the easier steps at the bottom rung of the ladder so that the steps become more and more difficult as you move up. You may also want to plan a reward to give yourself after you complete each step. Facing emotions that you have been avoiding is difficult work, and rewards can help motivate you to do difficult things. Your rewards could be anything from a special dessert to extra videogame time to painting your nails.

HOME LEARNING ASSIGNMENT

During each session of this chapter, you should continue to work with your therapist to identify an exposure you would like to complete for home learning. With each in-session exposure and each home learning exposure, you should be working up your Emotional Behavior Form so that you are exposing yourself to stronger and stronger emotions, without engaging in the emotional behaviors that are giving you trouble. Continue to track each exposure using Form 7.2: *Tracking the Before, During, and After*.

Remember that this is a gradual process, and it is not supposed to be easy! Try not to feel discouraged if an exposure is more difficult than you thought it would be, or if your strong feelings don't go away after you complete the same exposure several times. If your exposures are feeling too easy or too difficult, remember to talk to your therapist about this.

Also—remember your skills! If you notice before an exposure that you are having automatic thoughts that don't feel helpful or accurate, try to do some Detective Thinking. Or, if you are doing an exposure and you notice that you are trying to distract yourself from the emotion or situation, practice using the present-moment awareness skills. Try to use nonjudgmental awareness to be kind and compassionate toward yourself if an exposure doesn't go the way you planned, or if you continue to experience strong emotions.

Form 7.1: Emotional Behavior Form

Use this form to identify and describe situations that cause you to feel strong emotions, as well as the emotional behaviors you use in these situations. Using the Emotions Scale thermometer below, rate how much uncomfortable <u>emotion</u> you experience in each situation. When creating this list, think of behaviors like avoidance, escape, or other undesired actions (like aggression) which you may wish to change during treatment. As time goes on in treatment, you can use the last column (Did you work on it?) to see how much progress you've made on these behaviors over time.

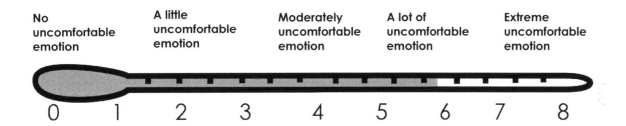

No uncomfortable emotion	A little uncomfortable emotion	Moderately uncomfortable emotion	A lot of uncomfortable emotion	Extreme uncomfortable emotion

Situation	Emotional Behavior	Emotion (0–8)	Did you work on it? (Y/N)

Form 7.2: Tracking the Before, During, and After

Each week, you will be asked to track the Before, During, and After of your emotional experiences. In order to change your emotional experiences, it is important that you understand the patterns that may occur (e.g., what triggers your emotional experiences, what happens as a result of your emotional experiences, etc.). This form will help you understand these patterns. By keeping this form and referring back to it later, you will start to see how changing one part of the pattern can change everything!

What happened Before? (What was the Trigger?)	What happened During? (What was your Emotional Response to the trigger?)		What happened After? (What were the consequences of your emotional responses?)	
	Thoughts	Feelings	Behaviors	Short Term	Long Term

Form 7.3: My Emotion Ladder

Goal: _____
_____

One Step at a Time:

Rewards:

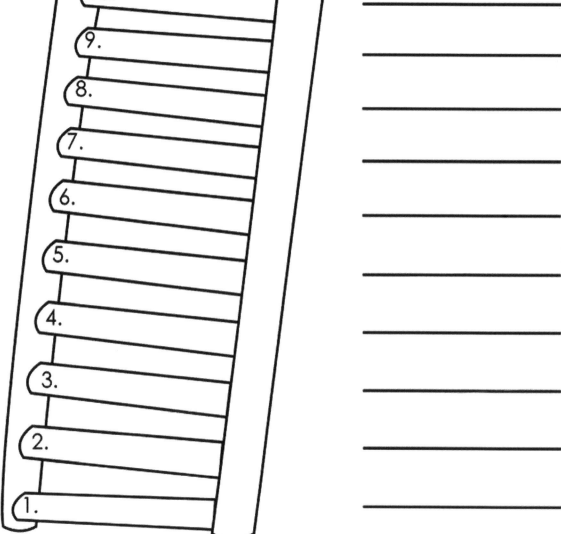

_____

_____

_____

_____

_____

_____

_____

_____

_____

_____

CHAPTER 8   Keeping It Going—Maintaining Your Gains

- To review the skills you have learned and practiced in therapy
- To celebrate your accomplishments throughout therapy
- To make a plan for coping with difficult or strong emotions in the future

Reviewing the Skills You Have Learned and Practiced in Therapy

Think back to the first session you had with your therapist during this treatment, and try to remember how you were feeling at the time. Which emotions were bothering you the most? What kinds of emotional behaviors were you using, and how were those behaviors causing problems for you? If you can remember, try to also think about how you were feeling about beginning therapy. Although some teens are enthusiastic about starting therapy, others doubt that it will work for them, think it will not be worth their time, or feel hopeless about things getting better.

Next, think about how you are feeling now. How have your emotions and emotional behaviors changed as a result of therapy? What is different for you now? How are you feeling about the future?

If you have noticed changes in your emotions and emotional behaviors, it is probably a result of using the many new skills you have learned during this treatment. Using Worksheet 8.1: *Skills I Know and How to Use Them*, take a few moments to review the skills you learned in each chapter of this treatment. Use this final session to ask your therapist about any skills you don't remember well or feel confused about. You may also wish to go back to some of the earlier chapters in this workbook and review skills you may have learned a while ago but haven't practiced recently. Ask your therapist if he or she thinks some of these skills are important to practice in the future!

Look through the list of skills covered in each chapter and think about which skill or skills felt most important and helpful to *you*. Take a moment to write this down, and then make a plan for how you will continue to use those skills in the future in your own life.

Celebrating Your Accomplishments Throughout Therapy

By this point in treatment, you have learned a lot about your emotions and how to cope with intense emotional experiences! By now, you have changed the way you approach emotions on a day-to-day basis using the skills that you have learned along the way. It is important to recognize and give yourself credit for all of the hard work you have done to make these changes. During session, your therapist will help you review changes in your top problems during therapy, as well as changes in the emotion ratings on your Emotional Behavior Form. As you and your therapist review these ratings, think about all of the areas where you have made progress. Maybe there are problems that felt overwhelming when you began treatment that feel more manageable now, or even problems that may have gone away almost completely. Maybe there are also situations that you can get through now without acting on your emotional behaviors. Looking at your top problem ratings, think about when some of these changes started to happen—was it after you began using a particular skill? Thinking about these patterns may help you and your therapist figure out which skills were most helpful for addressing which problems.

You should also note that most teens finish treatment with problems they still need to work on or strong emotions they still find difficult to manage. If this is true for you, know that this is common and try not to feel discouraged. On the next few pages, you will learn how to make a plan for continuing to approach situations that bring up strong emotions in the future, without using the emotional behaviors that get you into trouble.

Using Worksheet 8.2: *Taking Stock in All I've Accomplished* as a guide, think back on some of the most important experiences that you've had during treatment. Which skills, activities, or exposures most changed the way that you think about and handle your uncomfortable, intense, and difficult emotional experiences? Work with your therapist to remember your experiences and to recognize your accomplishments related to treatment.

Planning for the Future

As we have spoken about many times during treatment, emotions are normal, natural, and harmless parts of the human experience. This means that everyone experiences emotions, and even the most uncomfortable and difficult emotional experiences cannot harm us if we are not in a truly dangerous situation. This also means that you will likely experience at least some anxiety, sadness, anger, or other intense emotions in the future, especially during times of stress (for example, during standardized testing, when you have difficulties with friends, or when big changes—even good changes—are happening in your life). If you do begin to experience more intense and uncomfortable emotions, it is important to realize that this does not always mean that you are going to need to return to treatment. Rather, this would be the perfect time to take out your workbook and remind yourself of the skills that you learned in treatment.

Since intense and uncomfortable emotions such as anxiety, sadness, and anger are more likely to occur during times of stress, it will be especially important to remember to use the skills that you have worked so hard to learn and practice in treatment during those times. By now, it is quite likely that you have become such an expert at understanding and coping with your emotional experiences that you are pretty much ready to become your own therapist! Being your own therapist means (1) noticing when you are experiencing a strong or uncomfortable emotion, (2) identifying skills that would be helpful, and (3) making a plan to use them. Using Worksheet 8.3: *Becoming My Own Therapist!*, work with your therapist to begin planning for the future. As you fill out this worksheet, think about situations that still trigger intense or uncomfortable emotions for you and how you might apply your skills to cope with these specific situations.

Even though you will no longer be attending treatment sessions or seeing your therapist on a regular basis, you can continue to improve your ability to handle your uncomfortable, upsetting, and difficult emotional experiences. The key to this is continuing to practice your skills on a regular basis, even when you get busy or distracted and even if your problems may not seem that big. Eventually, many teens find that skills like Detective Thinking, awareness, and exposure become second nature to them, and they begin to use them quickly and automatically, without really thinking about it. You can achieve this too, but in order to get there you must continue to practice on a regular basis.

Being your own therapist also means living what we sometimes call the "exposure lifestyle." Living the exposure lifestyle means challenging yourself to approach situations that bring up uncomfortable emotions, big or small, in your day-to-day life, with an understanding that, while they can be uncomfortable, emotional experiences are a normal, natural, and harmless part of life. We want exposures to become a way of life for you, just like any other habit or practice you might have. This way of thinking about and practicing exposure may seem difficult at first, but with practice you will start to get the hang of it!

Worksheet 8.1: Skills I Know and How to Use Them

Below is a summary of some important skills you have learned in each section of this treatment. Take a moment to read through each skills summary and write down what you found most helpful about the skills. Next, think about how you could use each of the skills in the future. Are there certain times or places where they would be helpful? Are there skills you want to make a habit of practicing every day? If you see a skill you don't remember, you may want to check in with your therapist about it one last time.

Chapter 2: Getting to Know Your Emotions and Behaviors
Skills I learned: Purpose of emotions; Three parts of an emotion; Cycle of avoidance and other emotional behaviors
What I found most helpful:
How I will continue to use these skills in the future:

Chapter 3: Emotion-Focused Behavioral Experiments
Skills I learned: Acting opposite to my emotional behaviors; How to conduct an emotion-focused behavioral experiment; Connection between mood and activities
What I found most helpful:
How I will continue to use these skills in the future:

Chapter 4: Awareness of Physical Sensations
Skills I learned: Body clues for different emotions; Body scanning; Sensational exposures to stick with uncomfortable body feelings
What I found most helpful:
How I will continue to use these skills in the future:

Chapter 5: Being Flexible in Your Thinking
Skills I learned: Thinking traps; Detective Thinking; Problem Solving
What I found most helpful:
How I will continue to use these skills in the future:

Chapter 6: Awareness of Emotional Experiences
Skills I learned: Present-Moment Awareness (Notice it, Say something about it, Experience it); NonJudgmental Awareness
What I found most helpful:
How I will continue to use these skills in the future:

Chapter 7: Situational Emotion Exposure
Skills I learned: Identifying emotional behaviors that are a problem for me; Why situational emotion exposures work; How to do situational emotion exposures
What I found most helpful:
How I will continue to use these skills in the future:

Worksheet 8.2: Taking Stock of All I've Accomplished

1. What was the most difficult thing you did in therapy? How did you get through it?

_____

_____

_____

_____

_____

2. Do you see differences in how you react to strong emotions now? If so, what are they?

_____

_____

_____

_____

3. What would you tell other people your age who are having a hard time with strong emotions?

_____

_____

_____

_____

4. What is something you can do now that you weren't able to do before? What is something that you want to work to accomplish in the future?

_____

_____

_____

_____

_____

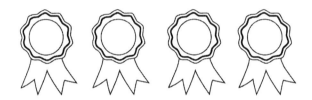

Worksheet 8.3: Becoming My Own Therapist!

1. What things or situations are still difficult?

   _____

   _____

   _____

   _____

   _____

2. How do you think you might handle these challenges?

   _____

   _____

   _____

   _____

   _____

3. What are the specific things that you are going to practice over the next four weeks in order to maintain your progress and keep working towards your goals?

   1) _____

   2) _____

   3) _____

   4) _____

   5) _____

   6) _____

   7) _____

Jill Ehrenreich-May, PhD, is the Director of the Child and Adolescent Mood and Anxiety Treatment (CAMAT) program and Associate Professor in the Child Division of the Department of Psychology at the University of Miami. In addition to the development and evaluation of evidence-based treatment approaches for anxiety and depressive disorders in youth, she is particularly interested in clinician training and the dissemination and implementation of effective treatments in environments that maximize their impact and benefit for children. Her current research has been supported by grants from the National Institute of Mental Health and the Children's Trust.

Sarah M. Kennedy, PhD, is a postdoctoral fellow at Children's Hospital Colorado, where she provides clinical services and conducts research on transdiagnostic approaches to assessment and treatment of emotional disorders in youth. She has published numerous book chapters and articles on the etiology and treatment of emotional disorders in children and adolescents.

Jamie A. Sherman, MS, is a doctoral candidate in the child clinical psychology program at the University of Miami. Clinically, she is interested in providing effective treatment for youth with a variety of anxiety and mood concerns. Her research focuses on the development and evaluation of evidence-supported treatments for pediatric mood and anxiety disorders.

Shannon M. Bennett, PhD, is an Assistant Professor of Psychology in Clinical Psychiatry at Weill Cornell Medicine, and is the Director of Psychology for the Division of Child and Adolescent Psychiatry. Dr. Bennett serves as the Co-Director of the Pediatric OCD, Anxiety, and Tic Disorders Program at Weill Cornell Medicine and is the Site Clinical Director of the New York Presbyterian Hospital Youth Anxiety Center. Dr. Bennett currently leads a research and clinical program serving children, adolescents, and young adults with anxiety and related disorders.

David H. Barlow, PhD, ABPP, is Professor of Psychiatry and Psychology Emeritus at Boston University and the Founder and Director of the Center for Anxiety and Related Disorders, Emeritus. He has received numerous awards and has published over 600 articles and chapters and over 80 books, and his research has been continuously funded by the National Institutes of Health for over 45 years. He is editor- in-chief for the Treatments *ThatWork* series of therapist manuals and patient work-books for Oxford University Press.

Made in the USA
Middletown, DE
10 June 2021